Strong, Savvy, Safe

*Empowering Tools for Self Protection
and
Vibrant Health*

John Pierre

Marina Alexander

Also by John Pierre

The Pillars of Health

In the Kitchen with John Pierre and Friends (DVD)

Vegan Weight Loss (DVD)

When Bachelor Meets Homemaker (DVD) with Dr. Kerrie Saunders

The Unprocessed 30 Day Challenge (DVD) with Chef AJ

The Ultimate Weight Loss (DVD) with Chef AJ

May this book increase your health, safety, and personal empowerment.

Contents

Introduction

What do you enjoy about life? Is it being with your children, family, friends, and animals? Is it surfing, swimming, golfing, or dancing? Perhaps you like to help others and feel great after watching their faces light up with delight and gratitude. Or maybe you simply enjoy breathing the fresh air, basking in the warmth of the sun, watching the seasons change colors, and seeing the birds and squirrels play outside in nature. As individuals, we all have different likes and dislikes, different goals and desires, and different perspectives. There are, however, some things that we all have in common: we're *alive* and we strive for things that bring us joy.

Unfortunately, there are those out there who wish to take everything that we hold near and dear away from us –including our very life. Their intention is to do harm to others for their own diabolical reasons and purposes.

To acknowledge that someone may wish to harm us and our loved ones–although we've done nothing wrong to them–is in itself difficult to wrap our head around. Agreeably, it's not the most pleasant of topics. It would certainly be far easier to pretend that the world is full of rainbows and lollipops, and simply push these uncomfortable thoughts aside; which, unfortunately, many people do all too well.

But choosing to ignore an unpleasant reality doesn't make it go away. If we decide to put on the mental blinders and shut down our awareness, it will allow us to pretend that we're exempt from harm. We then begin to exist in a dangerous state of denial; a frame of mind that discourages us from making serious attempts to dramatically increase our safety and the safety of our loved ones. And while we may live in an ideal neighborhood, have a generous bank account, enjoy a gentle-mannered spouse, and thrive within a supportive network of family and friends, are those things going to guarantee that nothing "bad" will ever happen to us? Realistically, who has the luxury of being that naive anymore?

What we really need, and what can truly help us increase both our safety and the safety of our loved ones, is to be stronger and more savvy. Thankfully, these are personally influenced qualities that we have direct control over.

With some dedication and discipline, we can work to increase our strength–both physical and mental–by improving attributes like balance, speed, coordination, and power; and increasing our overall health foundation so that we have a solid base to function from.

Being more savvy means we seek to increase our understanding, discernment, perception, and awareness about the dangers that surround us. The more knowledge we gain, the more solutions we can come up with to deal with various problems.

Acquiring practical skills and engaging in realistic training can help us shrug off those cobwebs of immaturity and blind trust; we can then empower ourselves with functional wisdom: intelligence and common sense that we can use for the betterment of ourselves and others. Why is that important?

Well, it's increasingly obvious that today's aggressors who commit harm are becoming more brazen and violent than ever. Just spending a day or two glancing over the headlines of our modern media, and researching the latest statistics on crime and violence will quickly open our eyes. During the research for this book, for example, it became clear that instances of violence were escalating and becoming so common and brutal that documenting even a small portion of them would take up all the space afforded here and more. Instead, an effort was made to intentionally omit a large volume of true stories to give the book a greater focus on practical ideas, common sense solutions, and valuable tools that can be implemented into a daily routine immediately. That doesn't mean that we're not metaphorically swimming in a sea of violent aggressors —we certainly are.

To our disadvantage, many assailants understand that they will not meet fierce and combative opposition because most individuals (particularly women) are not taught awareness techniques and vital self defense skills; making most people totally unprepared both physically and psychologically to offer effective resistance against any kind of confrontation—which is just how attackers like all of us to continue to be: weak, frail, and ignorant.

An environment where we lack awareness, insight, and effective skills to deliver effective opposition becomes a welcomed haven for violent aggressors who then gain the upper hand. Like an opportunistic deadly virus, assailants can and do devastate our society—if they're left unchecked. One of the goals of this book is to change that.

The information presented here may be an assailants worse nightmare. It's like having a manual that gives away some of the game plan—and that's the last thing an aggressor want's. It's not an overstatement to say that the knowledge contained in these writings may help save your life. This is a compilation of over 30 years of work and it's written specifically to empower you on a number of different topics related to your safety and wellbeing. And, while this book is written specifically with women in mind, anyone can benefit from the principles it contains.

These writings are concerned with saving and improving the most precious gift that you have—your life; while also increasing the safety of your loved ones: your children, parents, family members, friends, and neighbors. You will be challenged to take a closer look at your surroundings, your diet, your habits, your thoughts, and your beliefs; areas of your life where you may be vulnerable to attack—both from others and (unwittingly) from yourself.

Most importantly, this book seeks to develop your *survival mindset*: a frame of mind that cultivates your common sense, intuition, awareness, and every physical and psychological attribute that you posses. Because, with the right knowledge, desire, and commitment, helplessness and fear can be transformed into a more powerful frame of mind which can translate into actions that empower you on all levels.

You deserve to be healthy, happy, and safe. The aim of these writings is to assist you with these important objectives.

No Publisher Would Touch This Book

Let's face it, publishers are not in the business of printing work about unpopular topics, and it seems that the subjects of personal safety and empowerment are not considered hot or trendy—at least for now. The publishers who remotely considered this book didn't think the information presented here would "sell" on a level that would be successful, i.e.

that would make them a big enough profit. That's understandable since most publishers are in the business of selling books, not saving lives or distributing information for the betterment of humanity.

In some ways, this book is an antithesis to publishers aims because it's not written with the goal of making money or being on the best seller lists. It's goal is not to sell you any product or magic potion but *to sell you on your own self empowerment*. This is not a glamour guide that's filled with fluff or jargon, and it's not written for entertainment purposes. Like a true friend, this book is not going to tell you what you *want* to hear, it's going to tell you what you *need* to hear. There's a difference.

Telling you what you want to hear will no doubt make you feel temporarily cheerful and help you live in a fantasy world that's not based in reality. Telling you what you need to hear may make you slightly less jolly in the short term, but it will make you much happier in the long run. While this book won't increase your chances of getting a date, it may increase your chances of having a safer date or even surviving your date; and the only fashion advice it may offer you will be related to your safety.

Since one of the objectives of this book is to reach as wide an audience as possible with the goal of increasing individuals safety, those publishers who are inspired by the information found here are welcome to contact the authors.

What Does Health Have to Do with Safety?

It's sometimes easier to focus our attention on overcoming outside threats of violence, and ignore the many ways that we may be inflicting harm to ourselves. Sure, dangerous aggressors may hide in dark alleys, lurk around secluded parking lots, and hover behind street corners, but what about the most colossal potential assailant of them all—the one staring back at us in the mirror? While it's easy to point the finger at those who mean us harm, it's much more difficult to take sober responsibility for actively causing injury to ourselves.

It may come as a shock to you, for example, to discover that you may be causing damage to your health at least three times a day with the potentially deadly weapons called breakfast, lunch, and dinner; making detrimental choices and decisions—whether consciously or from ignorance—that may be wrecking the very foundation of your being.

The damage an attacker inflicts when he strikes may become clearly obvious very quickly, but it's often far less obvious to detect the harmful effects that you may be inflicting on your organs, arteries, brain function, and more, when you choose to ingest harmful substances. It may also be far less obvious to make the connection between your frail bones and the diet that you choose to consume. The point is that we can all unwittingly become our own worst aggressor if we're not careful, so the goal is to naturally take steps to prevent that from happening.

To leave out the health aspect and ignore it as an essential part of self defense would be to essentially disregard the very infrastructure of what self protection is built on. Many things in life work in very synergistic ways, and self defense is no exception. If the underlying foundations of your health are not sound, how well can you expect your strength, endurance, balance, critical thinking abilities, and intuition to perform for you when you need them to be at their most optimal?

Does it make much sense to increase your safety in some ways while you actively damage yourself in others? If you eat a diet that puts you at an increased risk of disease, and your bones in jeopardy of fracturing, don't you essentially injure yourself before an assailant even has an opportunity to get to you? Why help him do his job more effectively?

When you stop actively harming yourself in all ways, it becomes natural for you to want to prevent others from harming you too. Taking care of your health sends a message of love to your body, mind, and spirit that you respect and treasure them. In turn, they orchestrate their powerful efforts into giving you the courage, strength, and endurance that you need to defend yourself when your life is on the line.

How to Use This Book

This book asks that you consider the information presented in a fluid and flexible rather than dogmatic way. It offers adaptable concepts and ideas, not rigid doctrines that can't be modified to fit your unique situation. If the information suggests that you claw or rake an assailants eyes, there's no way of knowing if you'll really be able to do that in your particular self defense scenario. The attacker may be wearing a motorcycle helmet, making striking the eyes worthless; you may have a physical limitation or injury that prevents you from extending your arms, making striking the eyes an impossibility; and there may be other variables that may make striking the eyes of an assailant impractical or unattainable (he may be much taller that you).

So the best way to approach the subject matter here is to simply consider the concepts and ideas that it may represent. Ask yourself plenty of questions. Engage your common sense. Visualize scenarios in your mind. Spend time considering the information and pick out those elements that you find most useful and practical for your life.

While this book may cover a wide range of topics related to your health and safety, such a broad spectrum means that some subjects may be given less attention or simply mentioned to give you ideas that inspire you to research the information further on your own.

None of the material contained here will have any relevance unless you choose to integrate it into your daily life. For example, learning about and agreeing with the idea of keeping a map in your car is vastly different from actually taking the time to buy a map, study it, and have it handy in your car. Without your actions, the suggestions offered in this book will not become a part of your reality.

Neither will this book help anyone if it sits idle on a shelf. Consider passing it on or allowing someone to borrow it who may benefit from the information after you're done reading it. If you wish to keep it as a reference for yourself, then buying a copy for a friend or family member can make it a practical gift that may offer more value than clutter-promoting trinkets or gadgets.

To Health, Safety, and Self Defense Experts

If you're a highly accomplished specialist in some of the subjects covered here and you believe that you can add valuable insights to the information, you're respectfully encouraged to share your knowledge in a wider context. Please consider contributing your valuable skills, understanding, and counsel to others for the greater good of humanity. Safety, self defense, and health information that has the potential to save lives is too important to be held back from people who desperately need it; and we can all certainly use it now more than ever.

A Quick Word of Caution

The purpose of this book is to educate, and it's communicated with the understanding that the authors shall have neither the liability or the responsibility for any injury caused or alleged to be caused directly or indirectly by the information contained in this book. While the ideas described are based on common sense practices that are effective for over-all health and fitness, they are not a substitute for personalized advice from a skilled practitioner. Always consult with a qualified health care, safety, and self defense professional before beginning any nutrition, self defense, or exercise program.

Part I

Expand Your Awareness

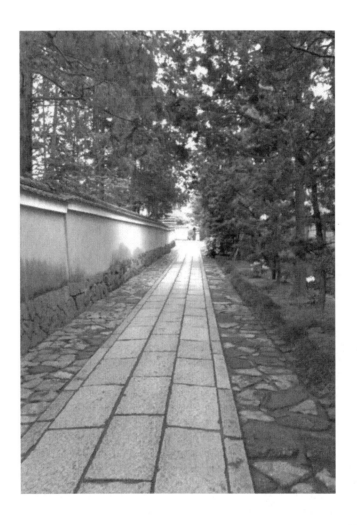

Chapter 1

Programmed Violence

Like the wind-blown seeds that fall and sprout in lush soil, the sights and sounds our innocent children see and hear take root and blossom in the fertile gardens of their minds. To put it less poetically: the sights and sounds our children get exposed to consistently have a profound affect on them over time. They help guide, shape, and influence their thoughts, feelings, behaviors, and ultimately...their very destiny.

We know that some proliferating weeds in a garden have the potential to choke and crowd-out the surrounding healthy flora, but what about the malicious seeds of glorified violence, destruction, and hate? If these "seeds" are "planted"–or programmed–in the minds of our vulnerable children, can they also become the metaphorical "weeds" that overrun, strangle, and obstruct the benevolent seedlings of peace, tolerance, justice, and compassion? And what kind of role does our modern culture play in encouraging violent behaviors? Could it be a more influential one than we may have imagined?

In the coming sections, we will look at some of the most detrimental "seeds" our modern society plants (programs) in our youth, and consider their effects.

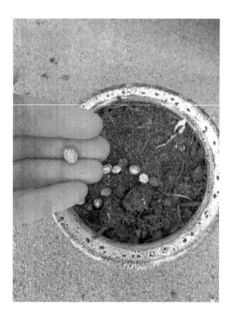

What kind of "seeds" are we planting in the fertile gardens of our children's minds?

Glorified Violence on Display

Television has slowly become the "filter" through which many of our human experiences are validated. This dark, square, domineering contraption, may as well be included in every house construction blueprint because most homes in our industrial society have one.

Today, television watching is by far the worlds most favored leisure activity.[1] It's so popular in fact, that American's over the age of 15 spend nearly three hours a day glued to their set.[2] It's reported that children in the U.S. watch 15,000 to 18,000 programming hours of television between the ages of 2 and 17; [3] comparatively, they clock-in around 12,000 hours of school during the same period, showing us exactly who the dominant "teacher" is in their lives.

A child's mind is similar to clay; it forms early impressions of what it sees and hears. This helps determine how a child will view the world. To the primitive part of our brain that's responsible for instinctual behaviors related to aggression, domination, and basic drives—*if it looks real, it is real,* because it can't distinguish between true reality and the simulated reality of television. That's why our heart starts to race and our palms begin to sweat during a scary movie even though we're only looking at a television monitor or a movie screen.

Television often exposes young, impressionable children to negative influences that may promote negative behaviors since its programs and commercials often show violence in a positive light. Children are shown, over and over, that aggression is the way to resolve conflicts. That's why, what passes for our children's entertainment today is often far from an innocent past-time. Increasingly, young children are indoctrinated from a very tender age to accept violence as a normal part of their recreation.

Children spend hours watching animated shows that often portray nonstop aggression from beginning to end —with characters inflicting mayhem to one other with dynamite, sledgehammers, guns, knives, baseball bats, light-swords, and much more. Often, the characters magically "spring back" to life after being destroyed. Shockingly, the rate of graphic brutality in cartoons far outweighs the rate of violence in shows aimed at the general public.[4] If we multiply the time children watch cartoons daily by weeks and years, we end up with an astronomical number of hours children soak up glorified hostility. Unsurprisingly, high levels of violence in cartoons can make children more aggressive simply because *watching violence influences young minds.*[5]

Viewing distressing scenes can leave a deep psychological scar and an invisible wound in a child which is not often seen or experienced until much later.[6] Violent content can induce fears and anxieties in children which fuel psychological trauma symptoms such as anxiety, depression, and post-traumatic stress.[7] Simply watching television during childhood and the teen years' has been shown to significantly increase the likelihood of people committing crimes, including *violent crimes*.[8]

With the unlimited supply of intensely gruesome and vulgar depictions hammering at our children's psyche from screens often located in the privacy of their own rooms, today's youngsters are at a greater risk than ever of becoming desensitized to violence.[9] Desensitization occurs when witnessing violence doesn't evoke as much of a reaction.[10] This may make children wait longer before calling an adult to intervene if they witness an altercation between their peers, [11] and results in a reduction in sympathy for the victims of violence.[12] We see this today when online videos show kids standing idly by watching and even filming school fights with their smart phones. Has their violent reality become just another entertaining show?

Naturally, television is the perfect medium for advertisers because they're well aware that viewers are induced into a passive state for absorbing information while watching it. So, along with the violent content pervading many children's programs, they may also be exposed to countless advertisements that contain subliminal messaging.[13]

During the past 40 years, an abundance of published information has surfaced suggesting that subliminal messaging can affect both adults and children's thoughts and behaviors—without their conscious awareness. In his eye-opening book, *The Age of Manipulation*, Dr. Wilson Bryan Key wrote: "Subliminal indoctrination may prove more dangerous than nuclear weapons."[14] Since we're not formally educated about the insidious use of subliminal's in television, movies, magazines, commercials, and billboards, the professional experts who make up the media industry can manipulate advertisements to their benefit with impunity by using undisclosed techniques–all without our knowledge, regulation, or oversight.[15]

Recreation or "Wreck-Creation?"

Some kids will happily forego the television if they're given the option to play video games. Suddenly, instead of being merely a viewer, a child can become an active participant who controls an animated characters every action, which is far more interesting and engaging.

Unfortunately, many of today's modern video games have morphed into something vastly different and far more dangerous than what children had access to decades ago and, of course, many are dominated by extremely violent themes. Violent video game "playing" can often morph into an insidious form of recreation, one that may be better described as "wreck-creation" because it has the power to plant the seeds of violence that program some children toward negative behaviors that end up inflicting lasting damage to them and to our society.

There's a reason our military has been using simulators based on video games for years to train personnel: the "games" ability to simulate real situations is uncanny. When we couple video games with a child's vivid imagination and his creative ability to vicariously project himself into the violent character's he now controls, the game takes on a "lifelike" quality.

A look at any child engaged in playing a violent video game tells its own story loud and clear: children's grim, expressionless faces appear robot-like, somewhat possessed, and partially hypnotized. Their hands are button-pumping away at the controller and their eyes are glued to the screen with laser-beam focus. Parent's who've tried to curtail their child's time from playing violent video games will often concur that they exhibit some of the same symptoms of addiction: irritability, lying, defensiveness, anger, frustration, and much more. Playing-time can quickly increase from hours to sometimes days; with some children missing meals and even showers to keep up with the "game."

Adolescent boys are generally the heaviest players of video games because many are designed to appeal to "masculine" themes such as fighting, sports, shooting, racing, or a combination thereof. Some games reward players with points for running over pedestrians, committing robbery, and even murdering a character. The winner is often determined by the accumulation of the most points. Shockingly, a number of video games have "secret" levels and "undisclosed rooms" which are not advertised and are unbeknown to parents. These hidden virtual levels further intrigue and mesmerize children to beat the game, adding to their appeal. Many kids end up sharing tips and tricks with each other to gain access to "rooms" where a player may have simulated sex or sexually assault a female character.

Unsurprisingly, studies have suggested that playing violent video games—especially for long spans of time—may increase physical aggression.[1] For years, the evidence has strongly pointed to the exposure of violent video games as a causal link factor for increasing aggressive behavior and decreasing empathy.[2] A recent study demonstrated that children with ADHD (Attention Deficit Hyperactivity Disorder) are especially vulnerable to the addictive use of computer games due to their neuropsychological profile. Playing video games for those who exhibit personality traits with aggressive cognitions, seems to further increase aggressive behavior.[3] Concerned teachers have also started voicing their concerns by stating that they now see some nine and 10 year old children in playgrounds display more violence after playing violent video games.[4]

What kind of "seeds" are violent video games planting in our children? Are the actions these games fostering helping to create positive or negative thoughts and emotions? If we consider that a recent edition of a popular violent video game grossed 800 million dollars in the first day of its release,[5] we realize that there are countless children (and adults) who are playing violent video games right now. This particular "game" allows players to torture others by "pulling out a victim's teeth with a pair of pliers, pouring flammable liquid over a victim tied to a chair, smashing the victims kneecap with a monkey wrench, and giving him electric shocks using spark plugs."[6] The back of the case reads: "Intense Violence, Blood and Gore, Nudity, Mature Humor, Strong Language, Strong Sexual Content, use of Drugs and Alcohol." Do you remember games like this being available when you were a kid? Is this kind of "game" content going to help or hinder our children?

Along with the violent media and video games readily accessible to today's youngsters, they must also contend with popular figures who may exude a dubious influence on their young, impressionable psyche.

Questionable Role Models

Not too long ago, many children looked up to their family or community members as their role models. Often, these individuals were not only personally known to the child, they were also greatly admired, respected, and revered. Because they exhibited outstanding qualities, talents, and values, they assumed a guiding role in a child's life; investing large quantities of time, energy, and effort in their wellbeing. And even though some mentors took on the responsibility of guiding other children, he (or she) still had a profound personal interest in each of the youngster's future successes.

In the past, this kind of mentoring process was instrumental in teaching and guiding children, and many cultures still sheltered from modern living continue to uphold this tradition. As the children begin to mature, their growing milestones are celebrated and clearly defined.

If we fast-forward to our modern way of living, we notice that many of our children's role models can now be found on television, movie and computer screens, CD covers, magazines, and billboards. The chances of a child actually meeting his idolized mentor face-to-face in modern times are almost zero. Because most of today's role models are "virtual," kids get a very narrow glimpse into their true nature and belief systems; and clearly, most "virtual" mentors have no personal stake in the success or failure of the children that worship them.

"Media mentors" are now commonly at the forefront of children's emulation because many kids hardly see their own parents, who are too busy working long hours just to keep up with the bills and the ever increasing demands of modern life. How many kids are greeted by a television set or a computer screen when they come home from school instead of the warm smile of a parent, grandparent, or other family member? Is it surprising then, that electronic devices—and the content that they push—start to become our kids dominating companions?

It would be naive of us to hold the belief that children are not being influenced into emulating the characters they see on TV and online—they definitely are. The kids themselves are not to be blamed—they're simply being programmed by what they see and hear. Youngsters look up to the personages in TV programs and reality shows because they're glorified in the media with attention, notoriety, money, fame, and power. They're talked about, focused on, and followed. Kids are frequently presented with a one-side-view of fun and glamour in the shows they watch, which can often conflict with the much-less glamorous, or sometimes negative reality of their own life.

So just who are our children's role models today? Well, they're definitely not based on the characters from the conservative sitcoms of the 60's and 70's. Children in our modern society emulate some athletes who use anabolic steroids and other famous performers who are morally bankrupt. Children's influential minds, without a consciously tilled path of their own, are influenced into wearing the provocative outfits they see famous girls flaunting on TV. They're exposed to simulated sex on television that leaves little to the imagination, which intrigues them into wanting to participate. They essentially try to be more like the famous and wealthy individuals that society says are popular and worthy of attention—because they want to be accepted and admired too.

Many well-meaning parents don't watch the same shows as their kids or monitor their activities online and have absolutely no idea who is influencing them. Even if television time is restricted, school provides the social environment where kids talk about the TV and online personalities they admire with friends; and many kids have smart phones with internet capabilities, allowing them to watch just about anything at any time.

One obvious solution is to provide a real-life mentor to a child. This could be a parent, grandparent, an older sibling, a trusted relative, or a close family friend who has high morals and values, and who will help support the child with care, understanding, and compassion. Children need a hands-on role model who's devoted to teaching them important life skills and attitudes that can help shape their moral character for the better as they grow. Media personalities certainly can't and won't do the job so the responsibility lies with us.

Inflammatory Lyrics

Words create vivid pictures in children's vulnerable minds, directly influencing their moods, feelings, and behavior. This means that those seemingly harmless lyrics they sing-along to countless times over weeks and months may be more damaging than we realize.

When children listen to music with violent lyrics, the repeating negative words play havoc on their psyche. Continually hearing the same homicidal words and sexual innuendos become their "musical mantras."

We've known for decades that emotionally charged words can evoke physiological signs of emotional disturbance.[1] When test subjects were hooked up to an EEG (electroencephalogram) and shown word lists with emotional implications, they exhibited increases in theta rhythms, heart-rate, and suppression of alpha rhythms similar to those of people under strong emotional stimulation.[2] If the listener of derogatory language trusts, believes, or identifies with the content (lets not forget that children are trusting and believing), then the *words gain an increased ability to directly and effectively control and modify his behavior*.[3] Of course, children naturally relate to the musical lyrics they hear because their glamorous role models are frequently singing the tunes.

Words have the power to make us laugh or cry, so it's no surprise that children exposed to parental verbal aggression become prone to higher levels of depression, anxiety, dissociation, and drug use.[4] When impressionable children become mesmerized by violent lyrics sung by their "role models," it becomes difficult for them to see logic and reason. If children spend time with peers who celebrate such lyrics, they often feel pressured to conform.

There are a number of violent genres of music listened to by kids today. The lyrics in some of these songs are filled with pornography, sexual assault, incest, sadism, and gruesome violence. Kids listen to and sing along to the inflammatory lyrics contained in the songs *all day long*. The performers of many of these bands appeal to kids because of their flashy jewelry, expensive clothing, cars, and perceived wealth. Kids then try to emulate these singers.

What kind of pictures are being created in a child's brain when he hears repetitive violent lyrics? What is he being brainwashed to marvel at? When kids hear that it's good to have sex on the first date, smoke and take drugs, and use prostitutes, do you believe this influences them to be kinder and gentler or meaner and nastier? Children who are susceptible to violent lyrics will find more reasons to accept the actions portrayed as normal and "cool."

What happens when a boy hears a girl being called a "ho" and a "bitch" in a song every other word? What is he thinking of when the song he's listening to talks about what a girl is going to do *for* him and what he's going to do *to* her in a violent way?

Listening to music with degrading sexual lyrics is related to advances in a range of sexual activities among adolescents.[5] If you're a young kid on the playground who listens to this daily, what do you start calling the little girls on the playground? You use the terminology you hear most often, especially when you think that it's "cool."

Many kids are singing along to derogatory language, shouting every adjective out-loud countless times —words that would never be heard on prime-time television. Violent lyrics and violent videos tend to bring out the worst qualities in people, especially young vulnerable children who don't know any better that they're being programmed for destruction.

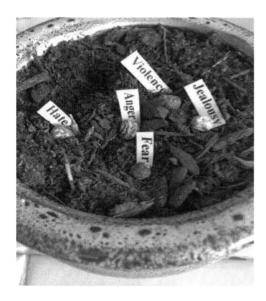

What's being programmed in our children's vulnerable minds?

XXX Seeds of Destruction

The following sentence will sound shocking to many
people, but it's a gloomy reality: Some of today's children
are watching pornography as early as sixth grade–and
they're not just watching two people having sex. Instead,
they're viewing an alarming amount of brutal and violent
pornography that's readily available online.

Just how easy is it these days for a child to take his
smart phone to class at school, put it behind his text book,
and watch porn while the unsuspecting teacher is talking at
the other end of the room about the ABC's? It's easier and
more common than we think.

Can we really believe that today's youngsters are
playing *Tic-tac-toe* or *Jacks* when they're out with their
friends? Do we honestly think that they're spending their
time drawing rainbows and unicorns? Hardly. Instead,
many children are spending countless hours surfing the net
because they have internet connections on their smart
phones or portable computers. You may be surprised to
learn that some of todays middle-school children are having
oral sex parties–children as young as 12! This is the
deranged reality we live in presently because our modern
society has insisted on continually bombarding youngsters
with sexual imagery that distorts their views of intimacy.

Of the two different types of pornography, one
particularly disturbing genre is called XXX (triple X).
These are films that display extremely brutal, vicious, and
abusive actions–movies of women being assaulted and
killed–often called "snuff" films. When children watch
violent pornography at a young age (not just sex), their
young, influential brain experiences havoc. The seeds of
violent pornography get planted in their mind and then

proliferate. Like a stuck recording playing the same song repeatedly, they may begin to obsess about the actions portrayed in triple X.

As children become more mesmerized by watching women being devalued and used as sex objects, *they stop considering them as human* any more. So, it will come as no surprise to learn that when children exposed themselves intentionally to watching violent X-rated material, it predicted an almost 6-fold increase in the odds of self-reported sexually aggressive behavior among 10-15 year old children.[1]

Another recently growing trend is that of high-school age girls who are being drugged or allowing themselves to get so drunk that they pass out while at parties. Unfortunately, some are then sexually assaulted by one or more assailants who take advantage of these girls coma-like states of unconsciousness. Since most smart-phones today have cameras, some guys have been taking videos of these unconscious girls while they're naked and posting them on social media websites to either brag about their criminal accomplishments or to further humiliate and demean the girls.[2] Sadly, not too long ago several girls have killed themselves after having this happen to them because they felt so humiliated.[3] It's a tragedy.

A 2010 content analysis of popular pornographic videos indicated high levels of aggression in both their verbal and physical forms. The perpetrators of aggression were mostly men and the targets overwhelmingly women. The women often showed pleasure or responded favorably to the aggression in the videos.[4] What message does that send to young impressionable children who watch violent porn? Pornography usage was further associated with individuals having more positive attitudes toward teenage sex, adult premarital sex, extramarital sex, more sexual partners, and engaging in paid sex behavior; i.e. prostitution.[5]

It's easy to think that just because we don't personally watch pornography that others don't either. The truth is that many men and teens (and some women) do. That means that the chances of us coming face to face with a man who watches violent pornography may be higher than we think. The person sitting next to us at the bar may have watched more violent pornography in the last few days than we've watched television in a month. The person driving in the car lane next to us may have watched several hours worth before stepping into their car. What's going on in their brain? What effect did it have on them? When a man speaks to a woman after viewing hours of violent pornography, does he talk to her spirit, her soul—or is he flashing back to what he just saw?

Women who interact with men need to understand that many may be watching violent pornography on a regular basis. Some men can "snap" when they watch it continually; it becomes like a negative affirmation that affirms violence and sadism. Triple X pornographic seeds create ideas and expectations that brew continually inside a persons psyche. Addiction to pornography is a very common obsession that can escalate to a desire to act out sadistic fantasies. Unfortunately, many aggressors are keen to use women and children for just such purposes, which is another reason why we need to be aware of the problem and be prepared to protect and defend ourselves and our children.

Lost Brain Function

Along with the violence-igniting sights and sounds bombarding our children, many of the "foods" consumed today are also highly inflammatory to their brain chemistry. Of course, the reasons for violence and antisocial behavior involve a number of factors and influences, but an often missing link is dietary nutrition.

It's well understood that without adequate nutrients, a brain can't function well. A poorly functioning brain has a difficult time using discernment and making good judgements. Realistically, how many children today are eating wholesome, unprocessed fruits, vegetables, legumes, nuts, seeds, and potatoes? The grim reality is that most are consuming sugar-laden candy bars, chemically jacked sodas, sodium-filled chips, and denatured cookies that not only contain little to no nutritional value, but many may also add to cognitive challenges; especially if they contain artificial colors and flavors (some are well established excitotoxins and neurotoxins), chemical enhancers, and rancid fats–which can play havoc on a child's brain chemistry.

The "junk food" diets typically favored by many youths today tend to make them more impulsive, irritable, aggressive, and sensitive to criticism.[1] A study performed by USC's Social Science Research Institute reported a strong correlation between poor nutrition, characterized by deficiencies in zinc, iron, B vitamins, and magnesium, and antisocial behavior.[2] It has been known, for example, that once a thiamine (one of the B vitamins) deficiency is addressed by supplementation, aggressive behaviors decline.[3]

Researchers have speculated for years that brain damage due to toxic metal exposure may promote aggressive, antisocial, and violent behaviors. There is evidence that aggressive behaviors may be promoted by the toxic effects of aluminum, cadmium, and lead. Lead exposure in particular has been linked with learning and behavior problems. The neurotransmitter serotonin has been found to play an important role in modulating aggressive behavior. The essential amino acid tryptophan is the dietary precursor to serotonin, and low tryptophan levels were found to be associated with high homicide rates.[4] There is additional evidence that hypoglycemia (low blood sugar) is related to hostile, aggressive behavior and a relationship exists between hypoglycemic tendencies and frustration and hostility. Since dietary sugar provokes insulin production which may cause reactive hypoglycemia, a reduction in processed sugar intake may reduce various forms of antisocial behavior.

Clearly, the standard fare being consumed by most children today is sadly lacking and far from sufficient in promoting optimal brain function. The coming chapters will provide information about empowering our nutrition to increase brain function, both for our children and ourselves.

Sedentary Childhood

Movement is critical to our wellbeing. The link between exercise and a variety of mental health benefits has long been established. Exercise spurs neuron regrowth, particularly in the hippocampus, a portion of the brain associated with memory, learning, and the regulation of emotion. So kids need movement for more than just their physical health; they need it for psychological stability and emotional balance.

But long gone are the days when parents had to call their kids in from playing outside. Consider just how often you see children playing, running, or biking in your neighborhood, particularly in groups, compared to when you were a kid. Many are now metaphorically chained to their television, computer, or video game console. Instead of playing in the fresh air and sunshine, our children are now bonding to their data-ports, which hijack both their physical stamina and brain function. That's one of the reasons that our children are now developing diseases that struck only the elderly in the past. Sadly, many of today's kids are engaged in a sedentary existence that sometimes rivals the idle lifestyles of many seniors in skilled nursing facilities.

Consider that many kids wake up after sleeping for around eight or more hours without much movement and then spend at least half of their day in school sitting down in classrooms. Some schools have made physical education (gym classes) a choice rather than a prerequisite so being active even for 40 minutes during school time is no longer a guarantee. When kids get home it's often time to eat and relax; i.e. watch television while sitting or lounging, text while lounging, or spend time on the computer while sitting. Homework is often worked on (by some but not all kids), followed by dinner and then commonly by more sitting and lounging. Unless the kids themselves are highly motivated to join sports leagues or engage in other physically challenging activities (either because they're internally driven or practically forced by their parents), many will simply avoid any type of exercise altogether.

This sedentary way of living deteriorates a child's nervous system while encouraging muscular atrophy and cardiovascular inadequacies. How many of today's kids can get up off the floor without much trouble? How many can do a pull up or a push up with good form? Children are also experiencing obesity at levels never before recorded in history due to a poor diet and sedentary lifestyle. Let's not forget that kids often like to snack when they watch TV.

Today's children (like many desk-bound parents) are sitting for prolonged periods of time, both at school and at home. This not only impedes oxygen delivery due to inadequate circulation but also suppresses the respiratory system. Their hip flexors get tighter and they may experience back pain.

Since automation is not showing any signs of diminishing (it's actually continuing to escalate at an unprecedented rate), if kids don't start to turn their sedentary lifestyle around it will continue to hinder their physical attributes and add fuel to the fire of poor health and cognitive challenges. The obvious solution is to encourage children to engage in physical activities outdoors and allow them to play outside in the fresh air and sunshine.

A Shift Towards a Brighter Future

When we consider the countless hours many children are exposed to violent programming through the channels of media, music, video games, and pornography, and couple that with a nutrient deficient and chemically filled diet, and a sedentary lifestyle (along with other contributing elements not explored in this book such as substance abuse, domestic violence, physical and sexual abuse, and more), we have an environment that's saturated with violence.

Of course, each individual is different and unique, and not all negatively violent stimuli will effect every person in the same way. However, some individuals seem to have an unexplainable violent "spark" within them, which our current society seems more eager that ever to provide the fuel and kindling for. An environment that's saturated with violence may provide the igniting elements that light that spark into a raging fire of destruction. That means that some people may get that extra "push" that propels them toward violent behavior from constantly engaging in violent video games, watching violent pornography, listening to violent lyrics, and eating a nutrient deficient diet, while living a sedentary lifestyle. All of these factors—to varying degrees—can help lay the groundwork for a potentially emerging criminal career.

Knowing that our modern society programs all of us and our children with dangerous "seeds" of violence should make us extra cautious about what we expose ourselves and our children to. Individually and collectively, we need to take responsibility and consciously program ourselves and each other with the valiant qualities of peace and compassion that we want to see mature and blossom today and in the future generations. If we want to see a brighter world without much violence, we can start to plant the seeds that take us in a better moral direction. After all, we can all use a better, brighter, and safer world in the years to come.

Take a look at the following suggestions to help our younger generation to attain more peace and wellbeing.

- **Create quality role-models for children**—Knowing how easily influenced kids are by "virtual" role models should prompt you to carefully asses who your kids are watching and spending time with every day. If you want your children to take on the qualities that are displayed by others, surround them with better role models who have high values and morals. People make a big impression in children's lives. Show them inspirational documentaries about real individuals who have persevered and overcome obstacles through high values, determination, and integrity. Remember that, as a parent, kids watch what you do along with what you say. You exert a great influence on them through both your behavior and your words. Model the behaviors that you would like your kids to display when they're older.

- **Play games with children that foster goodwill and cooperation**—Spend time playing games with your children that spark their intellectual and critical-thinking skills. Invest in board games, card games, and physical games (consider sports that you enjoy) that can be played while you spend quality and engaging time with them. Of course, video games that promote violence, aggression, and that demean and harm women and animals should not be on their list of pastimes.

- **Consider donating your television**—If you and your children are addicted to television and you can't curtail your viewing, consider donating your set to your friends or relatives for a few months. See the difference it makes in your life. If you feel that it's simply not for you, you can always get the set back. Try it and see what happens.

You may be surprised by the extra quality time you suddenly have to spend with your family.

- **Watch shows without violence**—If the thought of living without your television is simply out of the question, consider switching to shows without violence. This may be difficult to find but look for nature shows, documentaries, and educational and inspirational shows that lift you up and make you feel good. Game shows can be engaging to both kids and adults so look for game shows that you both enjoy.

- **Set parental-controls on your children's media devices** —Set parental controls on your children's smart-phones and computers so they don't inadvertently end up on pornography sites. Do the same with your television to keep them from viewing shows that promote violence. Be diligent about the social media your kids are posting and educate them about the predators who may be on the lookout for them online.

- **Know who your children hang around with**—Make it your business to know who your children hang around with, and the houses that they visit when you're not around. You can do the best parenting job in the world, but it only takes one of your child's friends to expose them to graphically violent pornography that may scar them for the rest of their life. That's why it's imperative to talk to your children ahead of time (keeping in mind their age and sensitivity level) as they get older about what they may encounter outside your home.

- **Make sure your children's diet is nutrient-rich**—You have direct control over what your kids eat at home so keep foods on hand that are wholesome and nutritious. Avoid buying and keeping junk food at home, where your kids will surely find it. Remember, their growing bodies need abundant nutrients, fiber, and antioxidants for overall health and exceptional cognitive function. The upcoming chapters on nutrition will give you a solid foundation which can be modeled to your children as well.

- **Create a supportive and nurturing environment**—Create the best environment that you possibly can to raise your child. Children crave their parents attention and affection more than they want fancy gadgets and gizmos. Those are only substitutes to take their attention away from what they really crave—your love. Yes, life can be busy and stressful, with constant challenges that take your time and energy away from your children. Let them know that regardless of how busy you are, you're doing everything in your power to give them the quality time that they deserve. Then follow up your words with action.

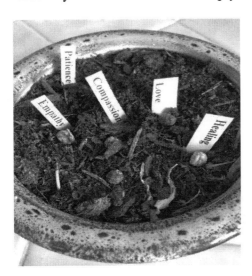

Our destiny and the future of the coming generations depend on what we "plant" in our youth today. Let's choose wisely, because we can all use a better, brighter, and safer world in the years to come.

41

Chapter 2

Identifying Malicious Intent

It's hard to believe that an important topic like predators is not a prerequisite study for adolescents and young adults in today's learning institutions. After all, they're taught about deadly viruses, dangerous fungi, and harmful bacteria, so surely they deserve to get a basic understanding of the parasitic aggressors they will meet in real life? Wouldn't such practical knowledge be potentially lifesaving too? Unfortunately, the subject is simply missing from the curriculum, which means that we have to search out the information for ourselves if we want to get an idea of what we're up against. Once we have that knowledge, we can then come up with practical strategies and solutions that will increase our safety. This chapter will get us started in that direction.

For our purposes here, a predator will be defined as any person who is causing or intends to cause damage to you or your loved ones physical, emotional, psychological, financial, or spiritual health. Throughout these writings, the word predator will be used interchangeably with words like aggressor, attacker, and assailant. If you prefer to use another word to describe the same genre of person for your own reasons, certainly feel free to do so. There are many to choose from, including but not limited to: psychopath, sociopath, bad guy, psycho, maniac, madman, creeper, nut job, or any other term that helps you get the picture.

Ultimately, the word you choose to use does not matter as long as it refers to someone who aims to or is actively engaged in causing harm to others with *malicious intent.*

Malicious intent encompasses everything that we could possibly think of belonging to the "evil" category: spite, jealousy, hate, rage, vindictiveness, meanness, nastiness, cruelty, and more. It's all the harmful things that we would consider a classic "bad guy" in the movies doing to others. Expect that it's real life.

Metaphorically, it's sometimes helpful to think of a predator as a virus that's programed to harm its host. To avoid the parasite doing us harm, we first gain a basic understanding of it's pathology. We learn what attracts it to a host and we learn of its own vulnerabilities. Once we're armed with that knowledge, we create an environment that keeps the parasite away; avoidance being our easiest and best line of action. But if the virus happens to gain a hold of us for whatever reason, our main goal is to get rid of the threat first, and quickly.

They Do Value You...as a "Target"

The first paragraph of the introduction to this book asked you to consider what you enjoy in life. After you read the short list provided, you probably had your own ideas to add to it, like vacationing in Hawaii, playing Frisbee with your dog, or watching your kids play a musical instrument during their school performances; joyful activities that hurt no one.

Predators are different, and so are their ideas of enjoyment.

As you've probably guessed, predators are nothing like the average, virtuous person—although they may look and act like one. Unlike the rules of fair-play, politeness, and consideration many of us adhere to in daily life, predators lack that critical moral compass inherent to most decent people. What were dealing with are individuals who contemplate ways of turning their violent fantasies into a horrific reality. These are people who obsess about ways to rip you off, use you, abuse you, torture you, assault you, assault your children, kill your children, and kill you. And that's just for starters. These actions may be on their enjoyment list.

Predators can easily harm others because they lack that critical quality that most normal humans posses: empathy. Without the ability to feel compassion and love, predators can stoop to levels of cruelty we may never fully comprehend. They get a thrill when they force, dominate, and instill fear in others. It makes them feel powerful. Some have had practice assaulting men, women, children, and animals, and have honed their "skills" over months or years. Their sadistic triumphs often inflate their egos and boost their confidence.

To believe that predators are less intelligent than the average person is the first mistake we make in underestimating them. Many are quite smart—they're just diabolically evil. They often think ahead, premeditating their actions and working out the details in advance.

Many aggressors are highly opportunistic and prefer to assault easy targets. In the scope of understanding their mindset, it's very important to realize that: ***The predator does not value you as a human being. He only values you as a "target."*** If you only get one takeaway from this section, let it be the sentence you just read.

Without the capacity for empathy or remorse, everything becomes just cold and calculated "business." Take out the trash? Check. Fix the car? Check. Mow the lawn? Check. Assault a woman? Check. Understand that predators see you as merely a *means to the end* they're looking for. Sure, no normal person thinks this way, but as you're now well aware, predators are not normal people.

Do predators know they're different from everyone else? Most likely yes. Many start to learn early on that what bothers other people has no effect on them. Watching the pain and suffering of others produces no emotion in them, so often, they learn to carefully observe the reactions individuals display to various circumstances; mimicking them to appear situationally appropriate. Mastering the art of acting early in life helps them fit in easier with everyone else, which is why it's often counterproductive to visualize a predator as some stranger with a gruff looking evil demeanor; most often look and act just like your average person. The difference is that they're not.

Since predators have absolutely no honor or empathy, and lack the basic human quality of caring, they will use all of our goodhearted rules of social conduct to their advantage. Unsurprisingly, many find themselves in high positions of power; working for institutions and establishments that seek empathy-lacking individuals to run the show. Since the valiant qualities of compassion, honesty, and fairness always put an individual's best interests before profits, money, and favors, these attributes naturally get in the way of a predatory-like agenda. Because predators don't posses these qualities, they have no problem using cutthroat tactics when they compete in the business world; and they can easily use their lack of compassion to coldly harm and damage others on a personal level, as they often do.

The ability to place ourselves in another persons "shoes" and feel what they feel is a natural human quality. When we see others sad or upset, it's normal to want to help them; to try to alleviate their pain and suffering. That's what makes us human. However, when a person lacks the ability to feel the emotions of love, compassion, and empathy, they essentially become more "robot like." This automaton-like behavior is typical of predators, especially when they drop their mask of pretense.

Naturally, our inquiring mind wants to know why people become predators. Are they born that way? Is it their home environment? Is it our culture of violence? No one can truly say. It can be a combination of all of these things and more. There are a number of theories that can take countless lifetimes to ponder over. Studies of serial killers, for example, sometimes reveal common factors that effected their early emotional development, including severe early childhood abuse, neglect, family addictions, mental illness, and even blunt head trauma. Other research sometimes points to the brain's chemical or biological impairment. And, of course, a violent media environment can sometimes provide the ideas and methodologies that can inspire a predator to become active. So there's no universally agreed upon reason that predators are the way they are; some spring up from good environments, and don't supply us with many clues about why they morph into dangerous aggressors.

At the end of the day, the most important realization to take away from this section is that a predator seeks to do you harm. It could be because of his genetics, biology, lack of empathy, boredom, sadism, or his drug-induced rage.

Will you really care what's driving him to attack you on some level or will you be more concerned about defending yourself and your loved ones? Will you be able to change a predators past, his physiology, or his bad brain-wiring? Can you instill the qualities of love or compassion in someone who doesn't have the capacity to experience them? Likely not. So your best strategy is to focus on the solutions that will keep you and our family safe from their attacks.

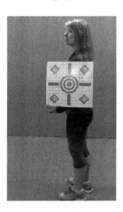

The predator does not value you as a human being. He only values you as a "target."

Just a Jerk or a Dangerous Predator?

Everyone can have a bad day now and then. Work demands, rushing to appointments, bumper-to-bumper traffic, and other common life stresses test the best of us to act calm, serene, and polite. That's why it's silly to assume that the next crabby person you meet at the checkout line, on the road, or at your friend's party is a predator. Generally, a very small percentage of the population are true predators. There is, however, an abundance of rude, insensitive, impolite, disrespectful, and ill-mannered people. You'll likely run into all sorts of individuals eventually, and a good majority of them, thankfully, will not be predators.

So how can you tell if he's a jerk or a predator? The following sections will give you some big clues. You'll learn how predators work to turn the odds in their favor and what aggressors look for when choosing a target. The information provided is meant to be thought-provoking; the goal is to start a dialogue in your mind that expands your awareness; to have you look at the common situations you find yourself in daily and ask yourself more questions that pertain to your safety. Every situation is different and unique. The suggestions and tips provided are general guidelines and suggestions that aim to spark your "safety-senses."

Are Your "Safety-Senses" Tingling?

If we study healthy animals living in their natural environment, we'll notice that they're very alert. Their ears are perked for sounds of danger, their nose sniffs for unusual odors, their eyes scan their environment, and they use all their keen senses to their survival advantage.

Humans are also naturally alert. We have a nose that picks up traces of odors that may signal danger, ears that are honed to hear the minute whisper of a noise, and eyes that naturally shift from side to side when we drive or walk to scan for hazardous obstacles. We also have a naturally keen intuition.

Our intuition is a kind of internal bodyguard; our built in red-alert system. It instinctively knows when we shouldn't be around a person or a place, even though we don't have a clue as to the reasons. We may sometimes say that a situation just didn't "feel right" to us or we had an internal "hunch" that something was amiss—and we're often right.

Although our brain can use all sorts of complex data to gauge a situation very quickly, our intuition is a kind of "knowing" that does not necessarily have logical origins. It may call for our attention with a pounding heart, sweaty palms, butterflies in the stomach, the hair standing up on our neck and arms, and a general feeling of unease which we can't verbally put a name to. It can pick up on a word or series of words, body language, tone of voice, or a change in facial expression like a smirk or grimace; and it can also cause us to hold tension in the presence of another person for no apparent reason.

Our unique intuitive sense has a particular feeling about it that we can learn to recognize. It's especially powerful when we can relax and allow our real feelings about a situation to come forward. If our intuition says: "This doesn't feel right," we should listen instead of trying to talk ourselves out it. Often, our mind has been trained to override our intuition by saying things like: "Oh, I don't want to be paranoid," "I'm over-thinking things," and "I'm just too worried," and we end up talking ourselves out of being more safety-conscious.

There are countless stories of women who diverted some disaster when they listened to their intuition. Sadly, there are also stories of women who chose to ignore it and the situation did not turn out well. Some women that have been interviewed by law enforcement personnel after they've been assaulted often state that they had an intuitive feeling that something was not right, or that the location felt odd, or that they really did not want to go somewhere with a person, but they fought those feelings and did it anyway. By then it was too late.

If we think for a moment about how an infant reacts to something that's bothersome: they don't ignore it and they don't "tough it out." Instead, they let us know exactly how they feel immediately. We're all born with this sense of self preservation, but most of us are quickly taught to distrust and ignore it. With all the constant distractions around us, we've become experts at overriding our internal warnings. Years of teaching ourselves to avoid our feelings, combined with our ability to numb them have deadened our most important warning mechanisms. This makes trusting our intuition a process that we have to relearn again.

The good news is that just because our intuition may have gotten rusty from disuse–like a seldom-used muscle–it can be finely honed to work in perfect condition; just like it was meant to. We simply need practice. It takes time to learn to listen to our gut feelings again. As we gain the trust in ourselves to follow our intuitive feelings moment by moment, things in life usually tend to go smoother. When we don't, we often end up feeling frustrated or depressed.

One of the aims of this book is to encourage the pairing of both your critical thinking skills and your intuition, and have them work together as supportive partners. While it's important to use your mind to logically think about potential safety risks in your daily routines and how to overcome them, your intuition should also be equally valued and honed to assist you in life.

Predator Tools that Smother Intuition

Did you know that there are countless predators out there who get together daily to talk about how they're going to assault a woman? Drugging a target is one of their easiest and often preferred methods of choice.

If our naturally keen senses, defensive cautiousness, and intuitive danger signals are lowered by drugs or alcohol, we not only lose control of our fine motor abilities, we surrender our capacity to think clearly, move efficiently, and in some cases—we forfeit our memories.

There are a number of very potent and easily attainable tranquilizers available today. Unfortunately, many often end up in a predators toolbox and become his favorite "tools of the trade." Commonly know as date rape drugs, these substances have been used on countless women around the world to invoke a catatonic state of immobilization.[1] Some women have been drugged, assaulted, and later woke up without remembering what happened to them because the drug induced a type of amnesia.

Date rape drugs are commonly dispensed to a woman when she does not have the physical or visual control of her drink—but these are not the only methods. There have been reported instances where men dropped laced ice into a woman's glass, for example, which shows just how devious these predators are.

Regardless of how physically fit we are or how impressive our skills are in the martial arts, these attributes will not help us if we're in a semi-coma from inadvertently ingesting a date rape drug—and none of our skills will help us recover from the subsequent amnesia. These drugs are very dangerous to our safety and should be considered extreme threats.

It's critical to be in direct control of your drink when you're in social situations. If a man you don't know brings you a ready-made drink while you're sitting at a table and asks to join you, be extremely cautious–that drink could already be drugged. If you order yourself a drink from the bar and sit your glass down to go dance for a while, consider that your drink may have been tampered with while you were away.

The most common date rape drug today, though, is alcohol. When a newly acquainted man buys a woman drinks, it's generally not because he's a generous person. Many men are simply using alcohol to "loosen" women up for what they're hoping will come later. Alcohol lowers inhibitions and predators are the first to toast, "Cheers!" when they're trying to get a woman "loaded." Once a woman gets tipsy, she become more susceptible and vulnerable to predators who love easy prey. "Ladies' Night" is a common gimmick bars use to attract paying customers (men) to a location that's packed with "loosened up" women. We don't see the sign "Men's Night" for obvious reasons.

It's becoming more common to hear about high school and college girls who get so drunk at parties that they pass out. A recent news story reported that a girl at a party became so unconscious from alcohol that the boys present were able to transport her to several different locations. They told people that she was dead because she was not moving, and took videos and drew graffiti on her body while assaulting her.[2] This is the sad reality when alcohol enters the picture; it's a serious drug and should not be taken lightly.

Don't fall for a predators favorite allies: drugs and alcohol. If you like to drink in public settings, avoid going alone. Ask a trusted friend or several friends, who will look out for you to come along. Make your safety your most important priority in social situations.

Retaining Unearned Trust

Would you allow a complete stranger to care for your infant? How about the guy you just met online? What about the "handy man" who just walked in to fix your faucet? How about your dentist, doctor, or priest? If you said no, why not?

Common sense dictates that just because someone appears to be safe-looking or has a "respectable job," that does not mean that they are good, kind—or *safe*. Convicted pedophiles have worked in some of the most trusted job positions, including priests. When a woman visits a doctor for a physical exam, there's a female nurse in the room present if it's a male doctor because having a title doesn't mean that a person is not capable of doing something criminal.

Some men start off acting as gentlemen, and end up exposing themselves for who they really are—predators. It's sometimes just a matter of time before the fake polished veneer wears off. Without a doubt, there are many men out there who are wonderful and kind. The key is to use discernment in weeding out the predators from the real good guys because sadly, many predators masquerade as gentlemen initially to get into your good graces, your home, your wallet, and sometimes—to your children.

The key to keeping predators far away from you and your loved ones is to work on building your awareness, intuition, and discernment. Predators can be charming actors, charlatans, and con-artists; leaving devastation, heartbreak, and ruined lives behind them. So it all starts with retaining your trust. As you've read, predators view others as being less than human. They look for opportunities to take advantage of women and they don't feel an ounce of guilt, remorse, or responsibility. Others use their work positions and uniforms to prey on unsuspecting and trusting individuals.

Recently, it was reported that a San Antonio police officer pulled over a young woman during a traffic stop; he handcuffed her, placed her in the back seat of his patrol car, and sexually assaulted her.[1] Sadly, this is not a random occurrence. Another report stated that a West Sacramento police officer was accused of assaulting six women during separate incidents by pulling women over while they were walking.[2] The truth is that a predator can be in any trusted profession and look like anyone. People that are placed in positions of trust violate that trust constantly and women need to be aware and alert for predators in "disguise."

Girls often grow up believing that certain jobs automatically command respect and indicate that a person is safe—a dangerous assumption. Women who were trained to trust unconditionally often do so, even before a man proves to be trustworthy. This line of thought is especially hazardous when a woman thinks that if a man's behaviors are good, then he is good. If he opens the door, pays for a meal, or gives her a compliment, it simply means that his manners are good, but it says little about his character. Good manners don't equal valiant morals and values.

Weeding out the Dating Charlatans

It's perfectly normal for women to seek healthy and supportive relationships. A growth-promoting, nurturing relationship can be a wonderful aspect of overall life-satisfaction and wellbeing; which means that dating is something that most women will go through during their lives—often, more than just once. Many will meet or be introduced to men who they may consider to be partner or "marriage material," but some, unfortunately, will come face to face with predators.

How often do young women receive classes on dating safety? Probably as often as they receive classes on self protection, i.e., hardly ever. So it's not uncommon for many women to jump in too quickly into relationships without fully comprehending who they're dealing with, which can sometimes end with heartache or worse.

Many men have a general understanding of women's "romantic notions," and they know how to play up to them—at least initially. That means many will be on their *best behavior* to look like a "good catch" or at least someone that a woman will want to get to know better. That man may be the most selfish and self centered individual anyone could ever have the displeasure of knowing, but he may showcase himself as an absolute gold-medal winner to get into a woman's good graces if he want's something from her.

One of the biggest traps women fall into is thinking that they will change the qualities they don't like in the man they're dating. However, reality dictates that no matter how kind, beautiful, talented, rich, or gracious you are, it's highly unlikely that you will change a man if he doesn't want to change himself. Consider carefully if you want to use your valuable energy on trying to change a man to your specifications. If he doesn't meet your standards now, chances are very great that he will not meet them in the future. Sure, some guys play a good act and change initially for show; most, however, go back to their old ways soon enough.

We often insist that manufactures invest in quality assurance testing for their products to make sure that what we're buying is worthwhile and safe, but how often do women put the men they date through the same rigorous examinations? Are some spending more time deciding what brand of face cream to buy than the man they choose to invite into their home?

Weeding out potential predators from the good guys takes time, patience, and many questions. Remember, unless someone is holding a gun to your head and forcing you to date; it's not a mandatory requirement, therefore you're in control.

When people first meet and are getting to know each other, it's perfectly fine to talk about the weather and common interests such as music, movies, and books. All of this information should be gathered in the public environments of restaurants, public parks, or other public places. Before you decide to allow a potential aggressor into your home and your children's lives, think carefully about the qualities they posses and if you've given them enough time to prove themselves. Remember, what's the rush really? Time is the critical factor in many cases, along with asking questions and receiving answers that are confirmed by seeing if the persons actions mirror their verbalized beliefs.

If you're in a dating situation or plan to date soon, consider making a personal list of questions that are important for you to know the answers to before you make a decision to get involved.

Red flags can be considered your built-in danger alert system that seeks to be listened to. They're often a combination of intuition, your biological sensory system, and a spiritually whispered warning. Consider some of the following "red flags" as a partial list of warning signals in dating situations:

Dating Red Flags

- He's *excessively* charming and complementary; trying too hard (above and beyond what *you* consider as normal behavior).

- He frequently glances at your cleavage or other body areas which *makes you feel uncomfortable*.

- He "accidentally" or deliberately touches your body in ways that *makes you feel uncomfortable.*

- He's willing to *drop everything* on his schedule to be with you at your convenience at any time.

- He speaks with hostile anger and resentment towards his ex-girlfriends/wives.

- He want's to start a family with you *immediately.*

- He makes exorbitant verbal claims of his financial success.

- He attempts to rush you into committing or making a decision.

- He stares at you in a way that *makes you feel uncomfortable.*

- He begins to insinuate or verbalize sexual innuendos to gauge your responses.

- He's *excessively* curious about your job prospects and salary.

- He *never* brings up his family, friends, or children.

- He's rude or obnoxious with the wait staff or the store clerk when he doesn't get what he wants fast enough or on his terms.

- He's aggressive, angry, and verbally abusive towards others–drivers, people in line at the store, and coworkers (guess what? You may be next).

- He's *excessively* inquisitive about your children in a way that *makes you feel uncomfortable.*

- He's *excessively* eager to baby-sit your young children when you're not around.

- Your own personal no-no's can be added here and the list can be quite long.

Note that many items on this list use the phrase: "*That make you feel uncomfortable.*" These are very important words. If something does not feel right, chances are that it's not. Use your intuition, listen to your feelings, and put the safety of you and your children before all else. Heed "red flags" and don't talk yourself out of listening to them when they pop up. Don't try to convince yourself against leaving a bad dating situation–it often gets worse, not better.

Why would you consider dating a man who sends out red flags? It's not like you're buying a used car that you can just "fix up," paint, and polish. People don't work like that so don't think that your incredible talents and skills will change your dating partner permanently into what you want.

Keep in mind that even if you do everything in your power to test out an individual as a perspective suitor there's still no guarantee. While most people can change with time, true predators won't change. Like a predatory virus, causing damage is their very nature.

If you're already in a relationship with a predator and want to get out, make sure you get helpful guidance, good support, and someone to help oversee your safety. This may include counseling, professional and legal advice, and safe housing.

Worthy Partner Qualities

The best way to meet wonderful and safe men is to stop wasting your time and energy on unfixable and dangerous individuals. Some women will keep tabs on the weather, what they have in the fridge, or how much gas they have in their car, yet many fail to keep a mental file of the character traits of the men they get involved with.

Ask yourself if you can visualize being with this person 10, 15, or 20 years from now. What does your life look like? How do you feel since meeting this person? Do you feel more grounded and balanced? Do your friends tell you that you've changed for the worse; being negative, distant, and aloof around them? Do you feel more depressed? Do you have trouble doing the things you used to do well every day like eating, sleeping, and keeping up with your daily activities? Are you picking up some of his bad habits, such as swearing or getting angry quickly? Your answers can give you big clues.

If your "safety-senses" are starting to warn you about a man that you've dated for a few weeks, don't continue to date him anyway. Recognize the problems you see before you, because hoping and wishing they'll go away is putting yourself at risk.

Get into the habit of buying your own meal during your first date. This lessens your sense of "He paid for my dinner, I owe him something." And even if you don't feel like you owe him anything if he pays for your meal, he may.

Take a look at the following qualities to keep in mind about a worthy partner. Continue to add to the list the qualities that are important to you.

- **Honesty**—This should be a given. Test for honesty continually when you're dating someone. How trustworthy is he? Is he respectful of your time by showing up as scheduled? Does his friends or family contradict his statements? Does his actions contradict his words? Place a greater emphasis on actions because, as the saying goes: "Actions speak louder than words."

- **Integrity**—Is the person you're dating willing to sacrifice something of himself for the greater good of others? This is a good indication that he will sacrifice his comfort and ease when you are ill or in need of help. Is he willing to assist in times of emergency like when you have a flat tire

61

or the flu? Test for anger reactions when you change plans unexpectedly because something important comes up like a sick child; is he sympathetic? Does he offer assistance or does he insist on keeping your joint plans for his enjoyment? Does he suggest that others come to your aid first so he doesn't have to? Test for integrity often.

- **Responsibility**—Taking responsibility for ones actions is a key indicator of maturity. Does he take responsibility for his actions, facing them head-on, or does he run away and shift the blame on someone else? Look for excuses that don't seem to justify irresponsible actions. Ask yourself how secure you feel with individuals who shun their responsibility. Do they command your respect?

- **Friendship**—Would you consider the person you're dating to be good friend material? If not, it can signal a real problem. If you're only interested in him because of his charm and appeal, remember that these can fade over time—while true friendship can last a lifetime.

- **Values**—Check for similar values. Does he believe it's okay to be with many different partners while you want a committed relationship? That's a recipe for disaster. Is he kind and giving or does he always want something back in return? Does he exude an attitude of: "What's in it for me?" Ask yourself if the values he holds dear are ones that you respect and admire.

Online Romeo's

In today's virtual world internet courting has gained much popularity; with countless women "dating" from the comfort of their own home. The occasional success story experienced by an online dating-service user is touted loudly in these companies advertising campaigns and commercials, but how realistic is that? Do you *really* know who you're conversing with on the computer?

A big part of how people communicate is based on facial expressions, body language, and voice tone—these are the main ways we show our emotions. Watching a persons facial signals can give us important clues and a lifesaving hunch about their true motives. Like a broadcasting station, facial features can shift in a fraction of a second to send messages about a persons emotions, mood, attitudes, character, and so much more. Many women are naturally accurate when making judgments about a man's emotions just from his facial signals, which give vital clues about his genuineness or phoniness.

When women engage in online dating, they can miss the subtle signs and communications that are crucial to really get to know a person well. When we read what someone is typing to us on a computer screen, our trained instincts—which normally look for facial signals such as a grimace, smirk, or smile—are not engaged and we can't distinguish voice patterns because there aren't any. Is the person on the other end giving us their undivided attention or are they "talking" with a number of other women at the same time? We won't know.

The danger with online dating is that we *think* that we know someone from writing back-and-fourth for countless hours. We invest time, energy, and most important of all—our emotions. Sharing our most private thoughts and vulnerabilities builds internal trust within ourselves with a virtual stranger—an individual we've never even met. Some women who finally come face to face with their "Online Romeo" are sorely disappointed when he does not meet up to their expectations, and these feelings may trigger depression and despair. Additionally, the man may feel as if he's "owed" something from putting in the time to get to know a woman. That can be awkward and may even escalate into an aggressive or stalking situation.

Obviously, the biggest hazards of online dating are predators, who are attracted to online dating sites because it gives them the ability to *camouflage* themselves behind a computer screen. Online predators can get a "lineup" of potential female targets and take their time studying and choosing a woman based on her looks and vulnerabilities. They can scope-out her weaknesses based on the words she uses in her descriptions and the insecurities she shares in her writing. The more self-esteem issues they sense in their target, the more they use those to their advantage.

Online predators may shower a woman with immediate compliments, praise, and "love"—feelings she may have never experienced around men. They can easily virtually seduce their target by conning her with false words and accolades. Since a woman can't see the online person in front of her, she can't distinguish his voice patterns, gestures, facial expressions, and all the other critical factors that are involved in finding out the truth about a person; and some women have inadvertently allowed predators into their life by way of their computer.[1]

If you chose to engage in online dating, avoid inviting the Online Romeo into your home and never give out your personal information. If you decide to meet the person you've been conversing with, do so in a public setting, preferably in the presence of other people that you know and trust. Online dating can open women up to potential predators who hide behind a key pad. Don't give them easy access to you and your children.

Creepy Stalkers

According to the National Center for Victims of Crime, one in twelve women will be stalked in their lifetime. Fifty-nine percent of women who are stalked are stalked by their intimate partner, and 81 percent of the women who are stalked by a current or former intimate partner are also assaulted by that person.[1] Unsurprisingly, 87 percent of stalkers are men.

A stalking may transpire over mere minutes or it may last for a number of years. Some stalkers make their intentions known right away and harass women with threats or lewd gestures while others may hide in the shadows without making their presence detectable for quite some time. Each stalker is uniquely dangerous situation.

Stalkers can break into a woman's car, house, or show up unexpectedly at her work. They can follow her to events, her home, and even stalk her online. Social media sites are particularly vulnerable to stalkers which makes keeping personal identity secure online critical.

A romantic relationship can sometimes sour into a stalking situation; a work colleague can turn into a stalker; a stranger who has set their sights on a woman turn into a stalker; a college classmate can be a stalker; a neighbor can be a stalker—the list is endless. Some harass a woman with intimidation, vulgar language, and threats.

Since many stalkers thrive on feeling empowered by their stalking, they especially enjoy targeting women and young girls who seem helpless, vulnerable, and prone to self-blame. Some women may feel too embarrassed to tell their family and friends that the person they dated or once considered a friend has suddenly turned into a stalker who now haunts their life. They may feel guilty about allowing such a person into their circle of trust to begin with, and not want to be seen in a lesser light by others for making a mistake.

Stalking can inflict untold psychological terror and fear on a woman who has to continually look over her shoulder and consider her every move. It's a type of psychological dread that tends to wear down a person over time. Common symptoms of stalking include fear, depression, nervousness, changes in eating patterns, loss of sleep, fear of being alone, and much more.

Support from family and friends is critical during these times. Women sometimes find comfort in joining a support group or similar environment where they receive validation and empowerment. It's imperative that you don't blame yourself if you find yourself in a stalking situation —it's not your fault.

Take a look at the following tips when dealing with stalkers. Some of them are taken from the *Victim Survival Stalking Handbook* (a valuable resource available free of charge at: http://www.stalkingalert.com/VictimSurvivalHandbook.pdf).

Tips for dealing with stalkers:

- If you're being stalked, don't keep it a secret. Tell your friends, family, and neighbors. Being stalked is not your fault.

- Consider telling your employer if you need additional security to escort you to and from your car before and after work.

- Report the stalking to the police and document every detail.

- Have a camera and tape recorder with you that's fully charged and easy to access. Most smart phones will have both built-in.

- Keep a diary of the stalking. Note the date, time, and location the stalking first started.

- If you see the stalker, be extra alert, and write down the date, time, and any other relevant details. Be sure you're in a safe location before distracting yourself with documenting the information.

- If the stalker is in your neighborhood, write down the names of any neighbors who may have seen him.

- Try to go out with others when possible.

- If you have a picture of the stalker, show it to the police, your family, and friends.

- If the stalker sends you a package, have the police handle it and fingerprint it.

- If you feel you're being followed while driving, go to the nearest police station.

- Keep any letters, notes, and presents that a stalker sends you (for documentation to be given to police as evidence), along with the date, location, and time received.

- Get the names, addresses, and phone numbers of any parties who may have witnessed the stalker make his threats.

- If the stalker is known to you, obtain legal council or speak with a police officer about placing a restraining order.

- Don't talk to the stalker on the phone. Hang up immediately. Note the date and time of the call.

- Don't erase a stalkers phone messages.

- Consider changing your daily routine.

- Change locks on your door and consider installing a security system.

- Consider keeping a P.O. Box and using that on your public identification (a good idea even without a stalking situation).

- Plan an escape route if necessary from your home or work.

- Keep yourself mentally strong and resilient.

- Focus on increasing your practical self defense skills.

- Don't allow a stalker to ruin your life. Being stalked is not your decision—it's not your choice and it's not your fault.

Energy Draining Predators

There are many ways to be harmed by predators, and not all of them are physically damaging. Beyond violence, predators can harm us in a multitude of ways, including causing an emotional trauma that might take months or years to recover from. Some predators are not physically aggressive, which means that it's very unlikely (although it's not impossible) that they will attack our body. However, just because they're physically passive does not mean that they're any less dangerous to our wellbeing.

Many emotional predators are cunning, manipulative, cold, and parasitic. Most know the difference between right and wrong but they simply chose not to apply that knowledge to their actions. Weeding out the emotional predators can be especially tricky because, unlike aggressive attackers who are immediately distinguishable, emotional predators often use stealth to blend into society, making them much harder to detect and avoid.

Emotional predators don't wear a sign that alerts you of their presence. They look just like anyone else, with the major difference being their inability to feel empathy. They also have a sense of entitlement to their presence which can often be mistaken for confidence. Since emotional predators feel that others "owe" them something, they have no problem in taking advantage of *anyone*.

While emotional predators may never commit an act of violence, they can be much more dangerous to our mental health, and the damage they may inflict mentally and emotionally can sometimes be worse. Physical cuts and bruises may heal over time, but the harm inflicted by emotional predators can last a lifetime.

A "psychic vampire" is a recent term used to signify a type of emotional predator who is extremely energy draining. Hanging around a psychic vampire over time may lead to nightmares, insomnia, poor health, and much more. They also seem to have an uncanny ability to saddle others with their problems because they refuse to take real responsibility for their actions.

Not all annoying and difficult people are emotional predators and it does not help to accuse the people that make you feel uncomfortable of being one. Some may simply be experiencing a bad day so it's best to avoid judging people we've just met because they may just be in a bad mood.

The key to gaining awareness of emotional predators is checking how you feel in their presence. If you feel drained, confused, and weary in their company and instantly feel better when you leave them, it's a good indication that being around them is not in your best interest. Unfortunately, it can be difficult to get rid of emotional predators because they tend to hand on like parasites. Many are experts at manipulation and pushing peoples "buttons."

An emotional predator may be a spouse who's verbally abusive one day and bringing flowers the next. They also excel at making people feel sorry for them—to their advantage. Since they're often driven by a destructive envy towards others, they generally enter into relationships of all sorts just to get what they want. Because they give nothing back and take all the time, the uneven energy exchange saps others energy, leaving them exhausted and confused. It's common to feel like one was metaphorically run over by a truck after dealing with emotional predators.

If you start to breathe deeper, feel better, and think more clearly when away from a certain person, chances are high that they may be an emotional predator. Sadly, most cannot be changed by others, so your well meaning attempts to heal and change them will often leave you in shambles—and them unchanged. It's best to remove oneself from emotional predators and warn others who may accidentally stumble into their traps.

Trying to help an emotional predator is often similar to pouring water into a bucket that has a gaping hole; no matter how much time, energy, love, and money you invest, it's never enough. You're left empty and miserable and they're only left wanting more. Take a look at the following partial list of tips to help you deal with emotional predators and listen to your inner voice if you encounter them.

Tips to deal with energy draining predators:

- Avoid emotional predators and refuse any contact and communication.

- Listen to your intuition and don't try to talk yourself out of how you really feel around a person who may be "sucking" you energetically and emotionally.

- Be weary of excessive flattery. Emotional predators can be seductively charming and often go out of their way to appeal to your ego in unrealistic ways.

- Emotional predators love the element of intrigue and drama. Do your best not to join them.

- Don't try to outsmart or psychoanalyze emotional predators–this will only drain you of your energy and vitality.

- Be cautious with your sympathy. If you find yourself pitying someone who is always hurting you or other people, and they are actively campaigning for your sympathy, be careful. Chances are that you are dealing with an emotional predator.

- Don't conceal an emotional predator from others just because you've been duped or feel embarrassed. Everyone deserves to be warned.

- Don't let an emotional predator ruin your life.

"Doormat Opportunists"

Do you easily give up your power and bend to the will of others, even if it's not in your best health or emotional interests? Do you often find yourself in situations where people "walk" all over you, and end up feeling like a "doormat" as a result? If the answer is yes, you may be creating a conducive environment for "doormat opportunists," who will happily benefit from your lack of boundaries.

Doormat opportunists are individuals who don't necessarily actively seek to harm anyone. They won't break into other people's houses to steal something, they won't wait around the corner for you with a baseball bat, and you won't find them actively looking to rip anyone off. They're not bad or evil individuals by any means, however, they can be lazy, unmotivated, and immature, which can make them draining to be around. They simply take advantage of an easy opportunity to slack off at another's expense and they use it as long as they can.

Generating a "doormat" environment is easier than we may think. In our quest to be kind, giving, and loving, we may have to find the right balance with doormat opportunists because they'll use all our kindness to satisfy their needs at our expense. We'll keep giving and giving, but there will be no reciprocation coming our way from doormat opportunists. And, if miraculously there is some return, the energy expanded by us to get it will feel more draining–like "pulling teeth."

Taking whatever others offer is what doormat opportunists do best, and they'll keep taking indefinitely if we let them. While energy draining predators actively seek to take, doormat opportunists will only take what they're given, without any malicious intent. The difference between the two is the intent. Doormat opportunists are often close family members and friends who use our sympathy to infringe on our time and energy. These are the "middle-age teenagers" who continue to have their ailing senior parents do their laundry, grocery shopping, and cooking when they're perfectly capable of living on their own and taking care of themselves.

The people around doormat opportunists often end up mentally or physically drained by overextending their time, energy, and vitality to those who have no consideration for others personal needs. It's a relationship where one party will often feel taken advantage of and used, which will typically damage their self esteem.

These are the individuals who refuse to take responsibility for their life, so they let others do the job. No matter how often we act to guide them with our time, advice, money, and helpfulness, they simply keep infringing more of their problems and dramas on us. They won't take our commonsense advice. They'll simply re-verbalize their problems to us ad nauseam. While it may not be in a menacing or mean way, it may nevertheless be extremely draining, specially if we're continually worrying about them or their issues. It's also disrespectful and unethical.

These are the people you wish would keep their business to themselves. Their conversations leave you emotionally overextended, particularly if you don't know how to help them. Sometimes asking the person to get professional help is the best option for all concerned.

There's a difference between being selfishly irresponsible and helping others solve their financial or romantic problems. When we don't allow capable adults to take responsibility for their actions and do their thinking for them, we rob them of cultivating valuable qualities and we often jeopardize our inner peace. This can lead to hidden resentment and disempowerment; uncomfortable feelings that cause many to seek solace in processed foods and other addictions for temporary relief.

If you wonder how you may have fallen into the dangerous and destructive pattern of being a doormat, consider that it may have occurred because you had low standards and personal boundaries. You may have also ignored red flags until the patterns became "normal."

The longer you violated your own standards and boundaries the easier it became to do it next time. You essentially trained yourself to accept the negative behaviors of others. Essentially, you taught them how to treat you. It's now time to take back your power.

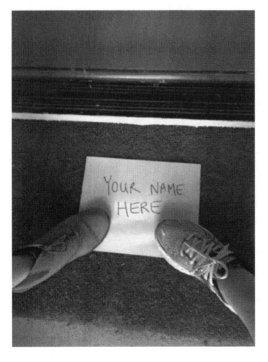

Do you often find yourself in situations where people "walk all over you," and end up feeling like a "doormat" as a result?

You help create a "doormat" environment when you:

- Allow others to treat you disrespectfully, even though you care for their needs.

- Take on other people's dramas and problems until they become your own.

- Take personal responsibility for other people who refuse to control their actions.

- Allow others to touch you in ways you don't like.

- Clean up other (capable) people's messes simply because they're too lazy to do it themselves.

- Do your capable, grown children's laundry, shopping, and more, simply because you've always done it and they're used to it.

- Put your needs and feelings last on the list and prioritize the needs of everyone else first.

- Hold yourself back from speaking out simply because you don't think you'll be acknowledged or treated with kindness and understanding.

- Surround yourself with people who don't value you because you feel that you're not worthy of better company.

- Wear certain clothes or a particular hairstyle simply because your spouse or boyfriend likes it–but you don't.

- Allow your grown children, friends, and acquaintances to have you on speed-dial when they want to vent their problems or frustrations, or need immediate solutions to their problems.

- Allow text messages at all hours of the day and night because others use you as a bouncing-board for their annoyances and every little irritation.

- Perform chores for other people but feel resentful about not being able to say no when you really want to.

- Allow others to be late constantly because they don't value your time.

Helpful Tips

- Teach the people around you that you are not there for their entertainment or to be used as a dumping ground for their problems. While you may be happy to assist and discuss matters, if their situation is very serious it may be more helpful for them to get therapy or professional counseling.

- Ask yourself this important question when you lean toward "doormat" behaviors: If I let him or her manipulate me right now, will they or I really benefit in the long run?

- Introduce your children or prospective spouse to the vacuum cleaner, mop, and washing machine early on. Teach them how to sweep, fold laundry, and pick up after themselves, so they're self sufficient and helpful; both for themselves, for you, and for the people they will be around in the future.

- Spend time developing your self esteem. Pursue classes and activities which uplift you and help you feel important.

Don't be Afraid to Say Goodbye

Imagine for a moment that you just got rid of a draining viral infection with hard work, time, diligence, and effort. You know it's going to take time to fully recover and begin to finally feel your best. So, would you consider allowing that virus back into your body? That would probably be the last thing you would ever want to happen. Yet many individuals allow predators of all sorts back into their life after they leave them.

Lets examine why.

The most common reason is that the predator temporarily reverts to their charming self and claims that they've changed. Yes, individuals who are not true predators—but are merely hurt or in need of healing—can certainly change, and we're not referring to those people. We're talking about predators here. They will not change.

It's common to also have ulterior motives of your own. A predator may have been supporting you financially, and now, without them, you may have to look for a job or a source of income that you have to provide for yourself.

This can be a scary proposition. It may seem that it's initially easier to get back with the predator knowing that he may be on his best behavior for a little while. That's entirely your choice. Simply know that your roller coaster ride of misery will probably continue. Do you really want to prolong it?

This book aims to give you tools of empowerment. Only you can decide to use them or not. Know that eliminating predators from your personal life is invaluable for your safety, self esteem, and overall life satisfaction. Whatever your personal weaknesses may be, focus on increasing your power and don't be afraid to say goodbye to individuals who cause you harm.

Chapter 3

Not an Easy Target

Predators are often sneaky and may sometimes stalk women or children for hours, days, or weeks before making a move. They also prefer "easy" targets because they naturally don't want to get killed, injured, or caught and incarcerated.

Knowing that a predator is looking for an easy target is powerful because it opens up more opportunities for us to make choices that stop triggering an "easy" signal on his radar.

You may intuitively recognize that predators pick up on nonverbal clues such as body-language, posture, alertness, and dress attire. Perceiving others is something that we all do quite naturally, it's just that in the predators case, he's using those clues to chose an easy target.

Consider if these signals have the same traits in common: distraction, inability to move effectively, loss of sight, loss of hearing, and lack of awareness. If you had to pick an easy target, would any of these traits show up on your "easy target" radar? Put yourself into a predators shoes for just a moment: What kind of target would you look for? Would the following descriptions make for an easier or more difficult target?

- **Talking on the cellphone while walking outdoors**—You send the signal that you're very distracted, not fully alert to your environment, easy to sneak up on, unprepared, and easily startled. If you must speak on your cellphone in a public setting, consider choosing a safe area where you can see who's around. Standing in a location where no can sneak up behind you is also very important since your focus is on the phone conversation. Be extra cautious when talking on the phone in public as predators can easily eavesdrop on your conversation and obtain too much personal information about you and your loved ones. An innocent: "I'll get Ally from school at 3," just alerted a predator that you may have a daughter of school age, her name, and the time you're going to pick her up.

- **Texting while walking outdoors**—Some people have walked into oncoming traffic, trees, and potholes because they didn't watch where they were going while texting. If all your attention is focused on typing words into your phone and reading the messages, a predator will see that you're distracted and not paying attention to your surroundings. Avoid texting in public and never text while driving.

- **Dozing on a public bus or train**—Sleeping while riding on public transportation allows a predator to scope you out and gauge your weaknesses or strengths without you spotting him. You advertise your exhaustion which signals "weak" to a predator. After all, if you can't even keep your eye lids open, how effective will you be at physically defending yourself? You may also miss getting off at your intended stop and find yourself in an unfamiliar area minutes or hours later. If you feel yourself feeling lulled while riding, try to stand up and hold onto something sturdy. Standing revives circulation and allows you to move quicker if the need arrises. You also gain a higher point of visibility from which to look around at others.

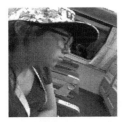 **Sleeping while riding on public transportation allows a predator to scope you out and gauge your weaknesses or strengths without you spotting him.**

- **Listening to headphones while walking or jogging outside—**How well can you hear what's in your surroundings if you listen to music as you're jogging or walking? Not very well. Why discard one of your keen senses when you're in public? A predator may be hiding in nearby bushes, ready to assault you just as you pass him. With headphones blasting, chances are great that you won't even hear him approach you. Avoid wearing headphones when you're out in public. Being alert to hearing an odd noise can buy you critical seconds to respond with aggressive retaliation or a speedy getaway which may help save your life.

- **Overloading yourself with bags or packages—**If you're carrying more than just a small bag, be very cautious as your hands will have to drop your articles to deliver effective opposition if you're attacked. Avoid carrying bulky packages which call for the full use of both of your hands. Be conscious about advertising the stores where you shop as criminals can deduce what price range you can afford based on the items sold in those outlets. Carrying bags from toy stores may advertise that you have a young child or children at home, even if they're not with you.

- **Wearing high-heeled shoes**—Have you ever tried running really fast in high heels? How about quickly moving diagonally or backwards? It's almost impossible to perform an effective kick to the groin or to an assailants knee while wearing high heels so be extra careful about the shoes you chose to wear, especially if you're going to walk alone through an unfamiliar area. Always keep a pair of sneakers or comfortable flats both in your car and in your handbag if you must wear heels to a special occasion. Change into your comfortable shoes when the event is over, especially if must walk to your car or another location. Effective running, kicking, and moving is critically dependent on the shoes you choose to wear. Put safety and comfort first on your list before fashion.

- **Dressing in constricting clothing**—If you're wearing a very tight skirt or tight jeans, how well can you kick or move? Can you knee effectively? Test your clothes when you consider buying them for your ability to move. When a predator looks at a woman in constricting clothing, he understands that she has limited her options in using her knees, feet, and arms. Let the clothes you wear add to your movement ability instead of taking away from it.

- **Advertising a hunched posture or depression**—If you advertise that you're depressed and hating life, a predator can pick up on those signals through body language. When you walk or stand hunched over and stare at one spot, you're signaling that life is not good, which gives the predator the idea that you have low self esteem. Predators know that a woman with low self esteem will have a lower chance of fighting for her life with aggressive conviction. Standing up straight and tall slightly increases your height and makes you look more alert. Make it a habit to check your posture often and send the message that you care about life and yourself.

- **Looking lost, confused, and unsure of your surroundings**—When you show your vulnerability to an opportunistic predator, he may use your confusion and need of assistance to his advantage. Be very cautious about approaching others for directions or assistance. If you're lost, pull into a gas station and go inside to ask the staff for assistance. Avoid accepting offers of help if you have a flat tire on the road or need additional assistance. Call a reputable towing service or AAA. Drive or walk to a well-lit and busy store and ask management for assistance. Predators keep their honed radar on women who look despondent and helpless. Be the opposite.

- **Avoiding eye contact**—One of the ways that animals assert their dominance in the wild is through eye contact. An animal that cowers and lowers their eyes shows weakness and powerlessness. Predators check to see if you make eye contact. If you make eye contact with a potential aggressor, don't be afraid to hold their gaze (without staring) confidently but not in a confrontational manner. Show that you are not afraid with your eyes.

- **The Fear Vibe**—Work on developing your skills and confidence with the suggestions offered in this book. This will decrease your "fear vibe," which predators look for when choosing an easy target. The more confident you look and feel, the more you'll be passed over as a too-tough-looking-to-take-a-chance target.

- **Letting strangers into your house**—When you let a handy man (stranger) into your house, you allow a potential predator into your home—and he didn't even have to break a sweat getting in. The same goes for dates. How well do you know your perspective suitor? Think hard before you trap yourself in a secluded place with a potential predator, be it yours or his. Arrange for a friend to be there when the handy man comes by or at least be on the phone and say: "Joe the technician is here now," or ask the man to speak quietly as you explain that your spouse is sleeping in the other room (to send the signal that you are not alone).

Consider Renting a P.O. Box

If you receive mail in an unlocked mailbox that anyone can access, how easy is it for someone to look through all your mail, and gain access to your name and the names of any other individuals who live with you? If your drivers license has your physical address printed on it and you lose it, whoever picks it up now has your photo, name, and address. How easy is it for that person to track you down?

That's why there may be benefits to renting a P.O. (Post Office) Box.

When you fill out forms and questioners, how many people look at your sensitive personal information or input that data into a computer? Do you know the individuals who have access to your physical address? Do you know if they leave your private information in full display of others, who may have ulterior motives?

Having a name along with a physical address gives potential attackers information about who lives at the residence. Does this woman live alone? Renting a P.O. Box, however, gives you move anonymity, which may put you at an advantage. If your correspondence and documents have your P.O. Box address, it may be harder to find out your physical address. That can put a little more arms-length between you and potential predators who may consider paying you an unexpected and unwelcome visit.

P.O. Box rentals are generally not very expensive, and their advantages may outweigh their costs. Yes, you will have to walk or drive to pick up your mail, but you'll have greater peace of mind knowing that people who see your address will not know where you actually live. That's priceless.

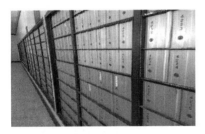

Renting a P.O. Box may give you more anonymity.

Secure Your "Safe Zone"

We often assume too much when it comes to safety. We assume that our car will be safe to get into, we assume that our work place is a safe place to be, and we assume that our home is as safe a place as when we left it. But bad consequences often come from making such assumptions if we're not careful.

How often do we get into our car without checking first if anyone is inside, or walk into our home expecting to enter a safe sanctuary; a place where we can finally relax and unwind after a busy day? Unfortunately, just because we step into the car or our home and close the door does not mean that we've entered a "safe zone" *yet*. The danger becomes relaxing too soon, before we've had a chance to check and see if our car or home is actually a safe place to be.

There are countless scenarios where aggressors may lurk inside our car or home, just waiting for us to arrive. In some cases, burglars are accidentally walked-in on as they're busy robbing the house, with them having no intention of harming anyone. However, that often puts them in an awkward predicament; they don't know if the person or persons arriving will do them harm, attempt to grab their stuff back, or try to keep them immobile until law enforcement arrives. All those are not ideal situations for thieves who want to get in and out quickly with their loot, so the arriving home residents may inadvertently corner these robbers into violence.

That's why you may consider it practical to check both your car and your home for hiding aggressors before you get too comfortable. How easy is it for an aggressor to break in to your car or home without leaving signs of forced entry, especially if you're not actively looking for them? Yes, you won't change the fact that an aggressor is already inside, but it sure beats being surprised by him when you're at your most vulnerable. In the case of your home, would you rather face an impending confrontation when you're fully dressed and on-guard or when you're coming out of the shower?

There's nothing unrealistic about checking your car or home to see if it's safe to be in before you get too cozy and lower your guard. After all, if you've been gone all day and the car or house has been empty, what guarantees do you have that others have not taken temporary residence there? Are they waiting for you and your family?

Yes, it will take a few moments to check your car, and a bit of time to check out your home depending on its size, but consider it an effort well spent. You'll notice if a window that you've left closed is now ajar. You'll also see other clues that can give you valuable information about the state of occupancy in your house.

Car and Home Tips

- As you approach your car, look for large vehicles like vans that may be blocking the view of your car from others. Consider if there are individuals hovering in the car next to you, and always carefully check your back and front seats before you open your car.

- Be aware that someone may be hiding under your car. Don't be afraid to slightly angle your head to get a better view of what's under your car as you approach it. If you see someone hiding under your car, immediately run toward a safe location and notify your local law enforcement.

- It does not hurt to check your trunk before you take off driving. Some predators have been known to hide in trunks and get out when you park your car in your garage; gaining easy excess, and a free ride to your home.

- As you get close to your car or home, check and see how you feel. Is your intuition sending you warning signals?

- If your dog is in the house, does he suddenly act strangely when you arrive? Is he running to a room and scraping a door while barking loudly? That can be an indication that someone is there who shouldn't be.

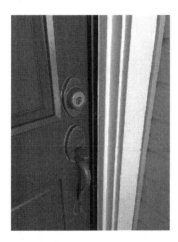

Get to know the general condition of your door. Spend time looking at the lock and consider what signs of forced entry might look like. Often, aggressors leave no telltale signs, so just because your door and locks look intact, does not mean that someone is not inside.

- Use your nose to identify any unusual odors when you walk into your home. You'd be surprised how often you can "smell" people who you don't know. It can be the smoke left on a persons clothing, a particular brand of soap he uses, the smell of inclosed spaces (like a car) where he spends his time, and other alerting odors of his cologne, hair shampoo, and laundry detergent that will alert you if someone is in your midst who doesn't belong.

- Teach your kids patience when they run to get into your car or enter your home. Avoid having them run into their rooms before you check the house. Teach them to stay close to the door entrance while you make sure that everything is okay. If you do find someone inside, they'll be in a better position to escape quickly. Train them to run out of the house at your command or if you don't return in a reasonable amount of time. Have them practice going to a safe neighbor or other safe location beforehand so they know what to do.

- If you detect any signals that things are not as they should be, exit the house immediately and call for law enforcement assistance from a safe location.

- If you park your car in your garage and use an adjoining door to access your house, be extra alert for anyone sneaking into the garage before the door closes, trapping you inside with one or several assailants.

- Don't assume that just because your spouse or roommate gets home before you that everything is fine. There may still be someone hiding in the house, waiting for an opportunity when you're booth asleep to launch an attack.

- Train your family members—particularly teens who often get home before you do—to check the house for signs of entry. Talk about the potential dangers of home invasion ahead of time, and come up with practical plans for your unique living environments.

Adopt a Friend

Assailants hate loud noises that alert everyone when they're around. The last thing they want is noise, commotion, and attention. That's why adopting a dog from your local shelter or the humane society may be the best thing you can do both for the dog and your home security.

Dogs are joyful friends who are eager to play, have fun, and brighten up your day. They have a keen sense of smell and their hearing is far better than any humans. Your canine friend's behaviors can also give you valuable signals when something is not quite right in your environment.

Just the sound of a barking dog can startle and intimidate an aggressor, making him think twice about taking criminal action. Barking is similar to having an alarm in your home which can alert both you and your neighbors of possible intruders.

Walking around your neighborhood (if it's safe) with your dog can sometimes be safer than walking by yourself. A possible dog bite is no laughing matter and will tend to give potential attackers second thoughts.

There are countless benefits that caring for your loyal friend brings; from daily outdoor walks in the fresh air that encourage your physical and mental health; to having the steadfast support of a lovable companion who's grateful to give and receive love.

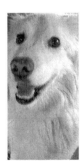

The physical, emotional, psychological, and *safety* benefits of caring for a companion animal are endless.

Chapter 4

Protecting Our Children

If you had rare and priceless valuables and a complete stranger offered to look after them for an afternoon, would you let them? If you said no, why not? It's reasonable to assume that you wouldn't have enough information about the strangers intentions, ethics, or morals, so you'd naturally want to avoid taking the risk of theft or damage. Sure, that's just common sense.

Interestingly, some parents leave their precious and irreplaceable children with strangers all the time. Many are simply too trusting and naive. They focus their time and efforts on color-coordinating their child's socks, buying them popular gadgets, and telling them fairytale bedside stories, but they don't consider taking on the tough task of educating their kids about predators; specifically, pedophiles who are actively seeking out young children for reasons of our worst nightmares.

As challenging as parenthood can be, single mom's often face even greater pressures from having to provide much of the financial resources needed to keep their kids warm, fed, and clothed. Unfortunately, single mom's are often on a pedophile's list of highly desirable targets. A single mom who's dating may run into men who don't want to get too involved with her just because she has kids—who they may sometimes refer to as "baggage." However, there is another category of men who want to date a woman specifically *because* she has kids. These types of predators are generally called pedophiles because they target vulnerable children.

A pedophile can use all his charm, appeal, and charisma to insidiously implant himself into a single mother's life, especially if he knows there is no other males around and she's eager to experience a life outside the home. Single mom's may have fewer financial resources and family support, and predator pedophiles can play up to those vulnerabilities by offering her money, a home, reliable transportation, and much more. Some single mothers's are often grateful for the attention, affection, and generosity coming from a man who they may see as their knight-in-shining-armor and another chance at romantic happiness.

Of course, not all men are pedophiles, as there are many good and decent ones out there. It may just be more difficult to weed out the predator pedophile because he may keep himself in "stealth-mode" for quite some time before showing his true colors. Sadly, a woman may never find out that the father of her children, her boyfriend, or her second-husband has been abusing her children for weeks, months, or years until after the fact. That's why it's a good idea to be aware that pedophiles exist and to keep your eyes open. This doesn't mean you have to be suspicious and mistrustful of everyone, it just means you need to be aware.

Parents should always be alert for predator pedophiles, but even if you don't have children; if you're an aunt, an older cousin, or have friends with kids, you need to also be diligent for pedophile signals so you can help those most vulnerable—small children.

One of the challenges with pedophiles is that many parents are not comfortable talking with their children about sensitive topics such as pedophilia. Kids don't need to know all the particulars, only their role in keeping themselves safe and telling a trusted adult if something happens. The more kids are educated about pedophiles, the greater their chance of recognizing the situation.

The problem is that this topic is often not discussed in families. Some women have been victims of family incest and never tell anyone because of self blame, shame, or threats. The pedophile often manipulates a child with threats of harm to her or her family. A male parent who is a pedophile can paint the picture of divorce, a broken family, or the damage to the other parent. And while it's uncommon, women can also be pedophiles, so leaving your children with a female is not always a guarantee that they will not be targeted.

Take a look at the following partial list of pedophile red flags which may warrant additional attention and investigation.

Pedophile Red Flags

- Listen carefully to the words your kids use when describing the man you're dating. Do they call him "weird" or "creepy?" A child's intuition is very high since it hasn't been stifled so it's wise to listen to what your kids say.

- It's a very bad sign when your kids avoid being around your date, relative, spouse, or friend at all costs—hiding or crying before he or she comes over.

- Be weary if a man insists that your child—who's perfectly capable of sitting without assistance—sit on his lap when there's plenty of other seating available.

- If he begins to buy provocative or inappropriate clothing for your child or insists on buying their undergarments you should be on "red alert."

- If he excessively showers your child with gifts, he may be trying to buy their affection or bribe them into silence.

- If you notice a change in your child's behavior after being around a person (this could be a male or female relative, friend, or date), this may be an indication that something is wrong.

- Most adults don't follow children around to other rooms or locations to avoid the prying eyes of others. Be conscious of the person who traps your child in secluded locations such as another room, the closet, a parked car, etc. What don't they want others to see or hear?

- Keep a close eye on any inappropriate touching disguised as tickling, horseplay, wrestling, etc. Many pedophiles create "games" that provide them physical access to a child's body, all under the guise of "play."

- If you notice that he dresses inappropriately around your kids (loose boxers with holes, loose robe without undergarments, etc.), it can either be a bad habit or something more sinister as some pedophiles are also flashers (those who exposes their genitals to others in public or private settings).

- If your kids tell you they're being shown pictures of naked people or someone is taking photos of them without their clothes, notify law enforcement immediately.

- If you notice unusual discoloration or dried fluids on your child's undergarments or clothes and you're suspicious about them, consider storing them in a sealed plastic bag until you find out what they are. If your worst suspicions are confirmed, this may be important evidence that law enforcement officials need to assist with prosecuting an offender.

- If your children tell you that they are being touched by someone on their private areas or that they're forced or tricked into touching others inappropriately, involve your law enforcement officials immediately. Pedophile offenders generally don't stop with one child. Putting a stop to their actions will prevent them from harming others.

- If you're not there—you just don't know what really happened. Listen to what your kids tell you.

Helpful Tips

- Educate your kids early about keeping their private body areas available only to themselves.

- Encourage your kids to tell you if anyone tries to touch them inappropriately. Warn them in advance that they may be threatened or bribed by that person but they should tell you anyway.

- Let your kids know *ahead of time* that if anyone tries to touch them inappropriately it's not their fault and they didn't do anything wrong.

- Alert the authorities immediately if you have evidence that you're child is being molested. Chances are high that they're not the only ones. When you stop a pedophile you help other children as well.

- Become aware of the sexual predators in your area. Online sites provide free information about sexual predators in many areas who must register with the state. It's a good idea to check anyone you're dating against this database, though it doesn't guarantee they will not be a future predator or are one who just hasn't been caught yet.

- Take extra precautions if you are a single parent who is dating. Know who you're leaving your children with. Would you leave this person to look after your rare jewels? If not, why would you leave your precious children with them?

- Even though you know and trust the babysitter, they may still allow other people into the house when you're not there. Ask your children if anyone else came into the house while you we're away (they obviously wouldn't know if they were asleep).

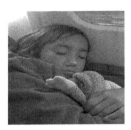 **Who has access to our vulnerable children?**

Additional Child Safety Tips

- Having your kids take self defense classes should almost be mandatory. Parents are hypocritical in some respects when it comes to making sure that their kids learn self defense. Mostly it's because they haven't been taught themselves as children so they can't be blamed to a certain extent since it's never been a focus in their life. Those that say they don't want to push their kids or scare them are doing them a serious disservice, similar to not teaching them to look both ways when they cross the road or warning them about touching a hot stove. It's never too early to begin learning proper body mechanics and movements that may help children escape by delivering an aggressive blow to a vulnerable body part.

- Discourage your kids from playing hand-held video games while they are walking home from school. This is just like walking with headphones on. Predators look for kids who are not paying attention.

- If you take self defense classes, share the simplest pointers with your kids and practice with them at home.

- Teach your kids about the targets and tools discussed in later sections. Use the functional fitness drills as fun exercises to teach your children practical motions. Kids will always be smaller in stature than most adults but their strike may hit an assailants vulnerable target, giving them time to escape.

- Make a game out of presenting your children with various safety scenarios and asking them what they would do in a given situation. Talk them through your reasoning process for the best course of action and be prepared to answer questions and discuss options. Take your time with these type of scenarios and start with the easy versions first, taking into account the age and personality of your child.

• It's never too early to empower a child with increased awareness, self defense skills, and an ability to think quickly in challenging situations. This knowledge may help them for a lifetime.

Family Escape Drills

There's a reason learning institutions perform emergency drills to prepare for fires, earthquakes, tornados, and similar disasters: they understand the value of practicing desired actions ahead of time, knowing that both students and school personnel will remain calmer when a real threat presents itself. Drilling a desired outcome automatically helps those trained responses to manifest during stressful times.

Considering that practicing in advance helps avoid panic, confusion, and lost lives, how often do you perform safety drills with your children in your own home? Sadly, many parents never even bring up the topic because they either don't think about it or the idea makes them feel uncomfortable. However, children have a natural survival instinct and they often listen to their intuition.When you couple these important qualities with practical and common sense advice, you train kids to look out for their safety and the safety of others.

Do your kids know what to do if there's a house fire? What about a home intruder? If you don't have a plan and actively practice safety scenarios with your family, everyone may be at an increased risk should an emergency occur. The time to discuss and devise a plan of action for keeping your family safe is before an emergency event, not during or after—by then, it may be too late.

Some parents think that roleplaying scary scenarios ahead of time will frighten their kids too much—but really, what's the alternative? Would you feel better or worse knowing that your family has a plan and some idea of what to do during a stressful or life-threatening situation?

Let's consider the scenario of a home invader. According to the U. S. Department of Justice, 266,560 people became victims of violent crimes during a burglary between 2003 and 2007. Sadly, households composed of single females with children had the highest rates of burglary while someone was present.[1] That means that home invasions are not uncommon. Some predators are savage and violent, and sadistically brutalize family members while forcing other family members to witness the assaults.

Kids don't have life experience, which is why they need to be taken through a role-play scenarios. Most children don't know what to do in emergency situations and tend to stay close to their parents for protection and guidance. But that may not always be the best choice of action. If an intruder breaks into a home during the night, a child may wake up and decide to explore the commotion, inadvertently running into the intruder and being used as a control tactic against other family members.

That's why you should spend time talking with your family about what they should do ahead of time. It's hard enough to make tough decisions in advance, let alone when you're awoken during the night, sleepy, dazed, and disoriented. If you train your kids to listen to your commands from another room and respond quickly, they will. If you role-play emergency scenarios with them ahead of time, you'll increase the chances of them responding accordingly.

Come up with a family escape plan and include your children if they're old enough. Have the adults in the household decide the best course of action, agree to it, and then present it to the kids in a serious, matter-of-fact way. The last thing you want to do is argue in an emergency about what to do. It wastes precious seconds that could mean the difference between life and death.

Home intruders have no qualms about grabbing a child and holding a gun to their head as they tell you what to do. They frequently go for the adult males first to incapacitate them to gain control. They count on your confusion, fear, and paralyzation. That's why planning ahead of time should always be part of your *survival mindset*.

Get your family together and tell them that it's important to discuss what to do if there is a fire, earthquake, tornado, flood, hurricane, or if an intruder gets inside your home. The adults should have a plan ready for each scenario and lead the discussion. If you take these scenarios seriously, your kids will too. Tell them their best options for getting out of the house. Let them know which escape routes are fastest for each room and why. Advise them where to run for help after they escape. Make sure they know how to use the phone to call for help and who to call, along with contingency plans if the phone lines are not working.

Children should know that they play a role in everyones safety, including their own. Getting actively involved helps them feel important and builds their self esteem. It's doubtful that there will be time for questions during an emergency. So when you train children to take practical and intelligent actions ahead of time you increase the chances of everyones safety.

Part II

Take Charge of
Your Health

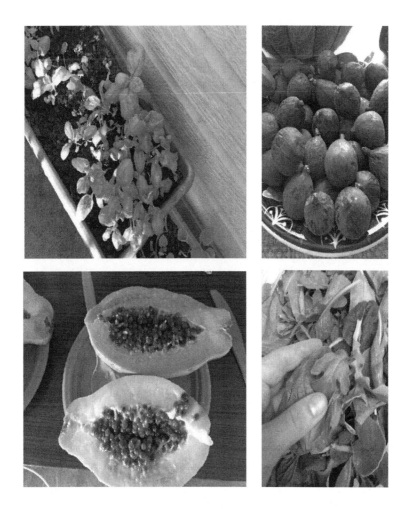

Chapter 5

Back-Stabbing Industries

Along with being surrounded by physical aggressors, we must also contend with other predatory entities that masquerade as indispensable product manufacturers. Some of these conglomerates require special awareness, attention, and discernment because they don't have our best interests at heart.

Predatory corporations excel at planting the seeds of discontent in individuals–particularly women–by showering them with unattainable images that are not based in reality. They disseminate the seeds of inadequacy and false promises, and keep people excessively focused on vanity and external appearances. Internal attributes of honesty, integrity, and moral values have no meaning in their world because these qualities cannot be bought with money. Their aim is to forever keep people focused on external distractions: the latest trend, fashion, sale-frenzy, passing gimmicks and more; downplaying meaningful inner qualities that are developed and cultivated with hard work, time, and effort–not questionable products.

Since there's big profit in fueling thoughts of inadequacy, individuals are often encouraged to tune-in to glossy magazines, infomercials, and mainstream websites for advice. But instead of getting unbiased, critically reviewed, and common sense data, some of these mediums of disinformation may provide a dangerous cesspool of inaccurate and corporate-influenced material that is likely to put our health and self esteem in serious jeopardy.

Just as cunning aggressors excel at hiding their menacing motives, some companies goals are also selfishly focused only on financial profits (less hidden and more obvious these days). Such corporations promote the instant gratification of every desire, often without question or contemplation. They benefit most when people feel dissatisfied with their weight, body shape, dress size, clothing label, hair thickness or lack of, and much more. They excel at flashy, eye-grabbing imaginary, slick photo-shopped pictures, and digitally enhanced depictions that expertly work to hook in unsuspecting "targets" (us) with the goal of selling their toxic lotions, harmful potions, and mapped-out fads.

Perhaps some of the most profitable corporations that hurt individuals today originate from the diet and fitness industries. These manufacturers create processed foods and other gadgets and gizmos that entice many unsuspecting individuals to join their engineered exercise frenzy. Instead of offering sustainable wellness, they give us questionable pills and diet shakes that often contribute to lethargy, poor health, and are the genesis of future diseases; conveniently failing to disclose that their nutrient-deficient and chemical-laden products often contribute to metabolic problems down the road. After all, it's in their financial interests to dumb us down with nutrient-deficient foods and to have us continually chase our vanity and ego.

If the fitness industry truly cared about individuals, would they continue to try to influence them to feel worthless? Why do some adolescent girls (who still believe in the tooth-fairy) feel inadequate? Because many have been constantly inundated with role-models who seem to have it all because of their appearance. These are often celebrities, rock stars, and fashion models shown on TV, music videos, and in magazines. The much less savory aspects of these individuals lives are rarely shown and are often downplayed.

When young girls buy into the fitness and diet industries hype and dramatically restrict their calories as a way of life, they often begin to suffer from eating disorders, low body fat, and amenorrhoea (loss of menstruation). Their hormones take a beating from a lack of adequate calories and nutrients some of these restricted eating plans advocate. The missing nutrients take a toll on their cognitive processes and invite Attention Deficit Disorders (A.D.D.), hyperactivity, and obsessive compulsive disorders. They don't realize that their unrealistic expectations are the result of the made-up ideals promoted and fanned by the fitness and diet industries. Some of these conglomerates have the power to help individuals, but instead choose to metaphorically stab them in the back.

Buying the "Skinny Equals Happy" Myth

Media conglomerates, with the help and patronage of the fashion, diet, and fitness industries have done a spectacular job of programming many people to center their thoughts around a very small and relatively insignificant aspect of life–outward appearances. Once our focus shifts and stays there, it becomes easy to buy the "skinny equals happy" myth.

Fashion magazines are now commonly portraying images that don't reflect real women in the world accurately. Many of their photos of women don't even look remotely natural anymore. Instead, their ideal female looks like she could blow away in the wind; without the strength or stamina to fight her way out of a paper bag, let alone do a push-up or a pull-up. They've created their own definition of normal: stick-thin; large chest; puffy lips; porcelain skin; an elongated neck; and very long legs. Of course, this is an unfeasible image of a plastic doll, not a vibrantly healthy woman. With work demands, family pressures, and so much more, how many women realistically look like this today, and how many are healthy and truly happy when they do?

Countless young girls and women aspire to be skinny simply because they've bought into the "skinny equals happy" myth that's been influencing them since birth. They want to look more like famous celebrities and highly paid fashion models they see in magazines, television, and movies, who seem to have it all.

Who tells women and young girls that celebrities don't look nearly as glamorous in real life? Does our media advertise the fact that some famous individuals subject themselves to surgical alterations, while others silently suffer from life-threatening eating disorders and exhaustive exercise regiments? Are we told that before these seemingly perfect women ever step out in front of the photo lens, they're clothed in expertly tailored designer attire to hide any flaws; and their professional hair and makeup teams put in long and grueling hours to make them look spectacular? Commonly, their best chosen photos are further photoshopped before they even come close to making it to print. How often do we get that information?

Advertising ploys often pay "lip service" to promoting real vitality and disease prevention, while aggressively focusing our attention on images of extreme thinness. Some individuals become so obsessed with that image that they become anorexic or develop other eating disorders.

If we take the time to look at healthy women in primitive tribes around the globe, we see that they naturally carry some body-fat and their skin appearance changes as they age. These are natural phenomenas that are nothing to be ashamed of, yet Tinseltown fairy tales try hard to convince us that they shouldn't exist.

In reality, beauty and thinness don't equate to lasting happiness and vibrant health; we're only sold the ideas that they do, to our detriment. If being rich, skinny, and beautiful were the real solutions to all of our problems, then Beverly Hills psychiatrist's offices would not be revolving doors for supermodels, professional female athletes, or celebrities; and no husband would cheat on his beautiful and very skinny wife. Yet many women still continue to be hypnotized, like the characters portrayed in the movie *The Stepford Wives*, to methodically get into the act of dieting; buying into the "skinny equals happiness" myth that modern media outlets gladly sell for their own benefit.

What most individuals really seek is happiness and love. Being a certain weight will never guarantee that we will attain what we want, but our personal empowerment can certainly put us much closer to our dreams and goals than what back-stabbing industries will ever offer.

Why Dieting Undermines Our Health

When individuals are enticed, coerced, or manipulated into losing weight, they typically start a diet. This temporary period of sacrifice and deprivation is familiar to many. As we limp through our restricted eating plan, enduring mind-altering cravings and hunger with steely determination, we count the days (and meals) until the punishment is over. Thoughts of food become our constant companions, whispering in our ear throughout the day.

Dieting often means we deny ourselves many foods (including important nutrient dense foods) for some time. It also assumes that we'll someday go off our diet...and then what? That's why the majority of calorie restriction diets today start on Monday and end by Friday. Eventually, most people are driven back to the food that they restricted themselves from. They also tend to gorge afterwards, which generally makes them gain back the weight they tried so hard to lose (plus some extra for good measure). Is that really a sustainable way to live and achieve health?

Unsurprisingly, most diets are not successful in the long term because they're not *lifestyle habits*. Even some people who've had liposuction eventually gain the weight back because the reasons they were overeating, along with their eating choices, have not been addressed. Going on a diet doesn't just magically enlighten us and solve all our problems; nor does it generally change our brain chemistry or overall health in a positive way.

While many individuals want to lose unnecessary weight, what they often really want to shed is unhealthy excess body fat. It would not be in their best interest to lose needed muscle and they'd definitely want to avoid dissolving their valuable bone mass—that would only lead to osteoporosis. And not taking in sufficient calories—which often equals less nutrients—is a sure recipe for muscle and bone loss.

Consuming a high-protein diet and enduring exhaustive cardiovascular exercise sessions can often spell a future health disaster. Many diet plans drive up our catabolic hormones and weaken our immune system, all while negatively effecting our cognitive function. Yes, we may end up "skinny" but we may also end up frail, weak, and cognitively injured. Who want's that?

There are more fad and gimmicky diet books on the market today than ever before, yet what benefits have they given us compared to the harm they've caused? Some people would argue that they create more problems than solutions because of all the confusion they promote about what's best to eat. A good majority don't even come close to touching on the real issues of just what went wrong in the lifestyle we were following to begin with; and hardly any touch on emotional and psychological issues that need to be addressed and healed before positive change can occur.

Some people that use calorie deprivation (starvation) methods to lose weight inevitably end up gorging on highly processed and sugar-filled foods that give the body a temporary high (which has been lacking for so long) followed by an inevitable crash. These crashes often fuel a catch-22 cycle—high sugar consumption followed by low glucose levels. This makes people just want to eat more processed foods. It's one big crazy roller coaster ride that's not sustainable.

Other individuals self-sabotage their nutrition goals on purpose when they see that becoming thinner did not solve their problems. It's a bitter pill to swallow when you learn that your solutions were within yourself, and not in your dress size. Often, the weight that was initially lost is gained right back, and the cycle continues.

Without real emotional work, which often ties into our spiritual and philosophical beliefs, it's difficult to build solid lifestyle habits that keep us on track to lasting wellness. The mental and emotional aspects need to be addressed too. Often, when we start getting in touch with ourselves again, we gain the ability to feel peace and contentment.

Diet plans that increase exercise but don't address the food aspects of good nutrition tend to lower calories, which makes people tired. They get so exhausted that they can barely do the exercises. That's like asking your car to drive more miles on less fuel! The coming chapters will discuss the best lifestyle choices that permanently build exceptional health–allowing you to leave dieting behind as a distant memory.

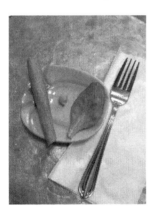

The majority of diets start on Monday and end by Friday because they're unsustainable.

"Scales are for fish, not people."

If you sometimes jump on your scale and find that your weight is down two pounds, do you ever wonder: *What exactly have I lost?* Is your scale intelligent enough to know the difference between your bone, muscle, water, and fat weight? When you retain fluid or build muscle, your weight will naturally go up. That doesn't mean you've gained fat.

If your goal is weight loss, the easiest way to assess your progress is to see how your clothes fit, how you look in the mirror, and how you feel and function.

Scales encourage constant fear and worry and set you up for disappointment. If you drink some extra water, this will show up as an increase in "weight." If you engage in strength training, this mechanical contraption will penalize you for gaining valuable muscle. Every time you look at the scale, you give away your power to a weight measuring device designed to keep you distracted with numbers rather than true qualities of health: high levels of energy, vitality, clear-thinking, happy moods, and the ability to move your body proficiently while engaging in fun activities.

That's why breaking free from your scale can be liberating on all levels: you'll no longer let gravitational readings dictate your very happiness; an imaginary number won't have the power to control your moods, confidence, and self image. Without the scale, you won't know the amount of "weight" you gain or lose—and you'll probably stop thinking about it altogether eventually. Your scale will fade away from your memory into distant obscurity, where it belongs.

Instead, you'll learn to listen more to your own internal voice that communicates what you really need in the moment—and you'll learn to follow it to your perfect health. Yes, you'll terrify the weight-loss industries who benefit from the constant fear and anxiety that scales promote—but you'll empower yourself to much greater life satisfaction and peace of mind.

Tricked into Guzzling Misery

It's sadly ironic that one of the most cruelly disempowering substances ever inflicted on humanity is so stealthily disguised and masterfully repackaged that it's hardly perceived or even recognized as being a threat. Through artful camouflaging and unlimited financing, the dairy industry has gradually hypnotized numerous populations into consuming their products.

For over 40 years, the dairy industry has used its bloated coffers to finance never-ending campaigns, catchy commercials, ginormous billboards, biased literature, and so much more to influence us into buying their products. They pay top dollars for A-list celebrities, child stars, successful athletes, and popular trendsetters to pose in ads with painted-on white mustaches to try to convince everyone (especially women and children) that they need a hormonal secretion that's found in a female cows udder.

In the context of human rights, everyone should be against cruelty inflicted on individuals—but what about the brutality that's forced upon living beings in the animal kingdom? The dairy industry has hoodwinked many people into consuming a substance that's not only specifically designed for another species, but one that also robs their health and desecrates the very spirit of female empowerment.[1]

The atrocities inflicted on a female cow during her lifespan can only be described as reproductive slavery. Milk "production" on many large farms today begins with artificial insemination, which can be more accurately described as sexual assault. First, a female cow is *restrained* and often put into a "head gate" or similar type of restraint. Then, an "AI" gun (an artificial inseminator) is *forcefully inserted* into her vulva (vagina), while the perpetrators other hand is simultaneously inserted in her rectum to feel out (through the walls of her rectum) the location of her cervix. The cervix is then grasped like a bar and the rod (Al gun) is threaded into and through her cervix, depositing the bull semen.[2] This is just the beginning of the cycle of suffering.

Similar to human females, a female cows gestation period is about 285 days (roughly 9 months and 10 days depending on the species). When a calf (baby cow) is born, his mother will naturally produce milk to nurse him. This hormonal cocktail is specifically designed to take her 70 pound newborn calf and help him grow into a 700 pound cow in less than one year—quite a feat! Feeding her calf by natures design is denied in most factory farms that supply dairy products to large supermarkets. Instead, either immediately or within days, the terrified calf is forcefully taken from his grieving mother.

Since a living, breathing female cow is merely viewed as a profitable milk machine, she's hooked up to a device which squeezes her mammary glands of her calf's intended sustenance, and her baby's milk is pillaged continually for human consumption. Many women reading this can well imagine the grief a new mother would feel if her child was savagely ripped away and stolen from her. After nine months of nurturing and growing a baby—the agony is unbearable.

Most female cows don't live long under the cruel and unnatural conditions of forced insemination (sexual assault), child theft, and milk robbery. The cycle of horror can only be repeated so often before constant stress, disease, and mortality sets in. The normal lifespan of a female cow is about 25 years or more, but that's drastically reduced to an average of about four years in the agribusiness-created model. When a female cow stops producing milk to their demand standards, she's discarded and slaughtered.

During pregnancy, a cow's estrogen levels skyrocket over 30 times higher than when she's not carrying a calf. When unsuspecting human children drink this hormonal concoction, their undeveloped bodies are flooded with estrogen and hormones that are both naturally occurring and those created by agribusiness. This sets them up for health disasters and social issues in the future.

In the not so distant past, girls didn't begin to develop until around the age of 15. Today, we're seeing precocious puberty at the inconceivable age of eight, which means girls are beginning to grow breast buds and will start to menstruate very soon.[3] When an eight year old girl who is pre-developing begins to dress like she's 12, she catches the eyes of much older boys who then begin to pursue her sexually. The consequences can often be disastrous: sexually transmitted diseases, teenage pregnancy, and sometimes even sexual assault.

Make no mistake—the most catastrophic substances you can possibly consume are dairy products. Cows are being fed bovine growth hormones to produce thousands of extra pounds of milk per year. These synthetic, pharmaceutically-made concoctions make a cows udders so distended that her teats drag on the ground. In factory farms, *there is no ground—it's called fecal matter or manure*. Dragging her udders through manure causes mastitis (udder infection) which often require dairy cows to be laced with antibiotics that end up in her milk.

Another dangerous constituent found in dairy milk is IGF-1, a powerful hormone. When IGF-1 is placed on human breast cancer cells, they grow like weeds, causing disease at an alarming rate. [4]Additionally, dairy proteins contribute to food allergies and autoimmune diseases, such as rheumatoid arthritis, asthma, and multiple sclerosis.[5] Lactose intolerance, the inability to digest the milk sugar lactose, is often responsible for stomach cramps, bloating, gas, and diarrhea.

Most cows in factory farms are being fed genetically modified grains that are also contaminated with unregulated pesticides. Since cows eat massive amounts of toxic grains over their lifespan, when human children drink body fluids from dairy cows, the residue of poison is delivered to them in a *concentrated* form. What are we setting children up for when we insist that they drink cow's milk?

The consequences of dairy products are easy to distinguish: precocious puberty, frail bones, obesity, heart disease, stroke, arthritis, diabetes, and the cruelty inflicted upon a species that continues to suffer. Sadly, the dairy industry has programmed many individuals to fear going without their products by fueling a society-wide calcium anxiety, which will be discussed next.

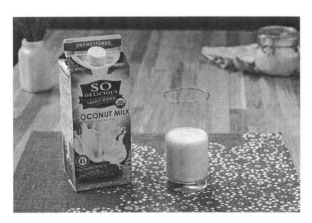

It's easier than ever to give up dairy products and embrace delicious alternatives that can be used in many recipes as well.

Engineered Osteoporosis Phobia

Along with being denied the real information about the inescapable cruelty found in every drop of cows milk, many individuals have been additionally brainwashed by the dairy industry into believing that they need large amounts of calcium for their bones. A popular trick-of-the-trade is to use scare tactics that frighten people (particularly women) into consuming their products–which in itself should set off alarm bells.

Fear is a powerful sales-weapon, and the dairy industry puts it to expert use by throwing big money at marketing campaigns designed to push the idea that individuals must consume their products or suffer the devastating consequences of osteoporosis. But, if that was really the case, how did countless civilizations thrive and flourish for eons without a drop of cows "ivory syrup?" Many populations around the world have never even seen a cow, let alone drank her hormonal secretions, all while enjoying exceptional health and longevity.

Bone is a living tissue that grows, repairs, and renews itself throughout our life. Osteoporosis is a condition where bones lose mass, weaken, and become susceptible to fracture. Adequate bone health requires far more nutrients than just calcium. Others include boron, vitamin D, vitamin K, vitamin C, zinc, and more. There are a number of negative factors that contribute to bone loss; including: refined sugar, salt, caffeine, nicotine, and phosphoric acid (an additive in some sodas). A sedentary lifestyle also increases the rate of calcium loss. Exercise, particularly weight bearing exercise, helps increase bone mass and may reverse bone loss. Bone-building exercise contributes to the development and growth of bone tissue (many of the movements introduced in the coming sections help develop bone density).

Preventing and successfully treating osteoporosis starts with plants and bone-building exercises. Plants absorb calcium and other minerals from the soil, which are then built into their roots and stems. The best sources of minerals are green vegetables such as broccoli, chard, and kale; along with whole grains, beans, nuts, seeds, and sea vegetables.

There's no need to buy into the dairy industry hype and have an osteoporosis-phobia. Simply eat an adequate supply of fruits, vegetables, whole grains, tubers, and legumes, along with small amounts of nuts and seeds, and engage in sufficient movement over the course of your day to stimulate the growth of bone tissue. It's easy to leave the calcium fears behind, and the following chapters will show you how a good nutrition foundation will help build not only strong bones, but lasting wellbeing.

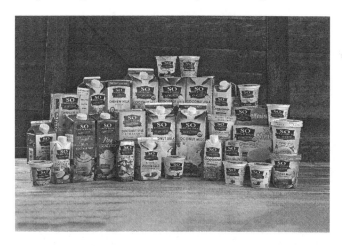

Companies such as So Delicious Dairy Free have helped countless individuals embrace a dairy free lifestyle by offering a wide variety of products that invite people to make the transition easily and effortlessly.

Programmed Protein Anxiety

Perhaps the most controversial and misunderstood topic in the field of nutrition is protein. Despite proteins top-stage presence in many articles, the average person can't name exactly what protein is and what it does. All they know is what they heard someone else mention or a quick headline that made things even more confusing. That's understandable since we've been completely inundated by conflicting information in this area, so the majority of individuals are under intentionally false impressions about this macronutrient.

The basic description of protein is that it's a nutrient that's needed to build, maintain, and repair body tissues. While we've been influenced to believe that we need a great deal of protein to thrive, quite the opposite is true. Our highest requirement for protein is during infancy, when the average baby is growing the fastest. Surprisingly, human mothers breast milk is only about 4-5% protein. Nature is incredibly smart and knows what to do. If not, would we have made it as a species this long on this planet? After we're weaned from our mothers milk (between the ages of 2-4) most people gradually lose the ability to digest milk because many gradually lose the ability to produce the enzymes necessary for its digestion. We continue growing but receive the nourishment we need from solid foods; as nature designed our system to eat solid foods after we stop suckling.

It was once thought that plant proteins were "incomplete," meaning, they did not posses all the essential amino acids that animal flesh foods contained. We now know that this is not how the body uses amino acids. In its infinite wisdom, our body patiently waits until it receives various amino acids at different time frames. Then, it assembles, stores, and combines them to make complete protein. Foods containing some amino acids but not others do not have to be eaten together at the same time to make this work. Think of amino acids as letters that make complete words. All foods have various letters and the body knows which ones it needs to make complete words and sentences. As long as we eat a wide variety of whole foods, our body will be able to build those sentences effectively. If we look at the biggest animals in nature, whether it's the elephant or the silverback gorilla, we see that they are not eating so called "complete" proteins. They are just eating a variety of foods all the time.

We rarely find documented cases of protein deficiency in America. It's theoretically only possible if we do not consume adequate calories to sustain life, but then −we'd be deficient in just about everything, including protein. The Recommended Dietary Allowance (RDA) for protein for the average adult is about 0.8 grams per kilogram of body weight. One kilogram is .453 of a pound. This means that a person who is 125 pounds needs about 56 grams of protein daily. Remember, this is a generous number that is designed to overcompensate for any possible protein deficiency. These 56 grams can be easily accomplished by eating 1/2 cup of tofu (20 grams), 1 cup of black beans (15 grams), 1 cup of quinoa (11 grams) and 2 1/4 cups of broccoli (10 grams). What's great about eating these foods is that they are filled with nutrients and fiber.

Animal flesh foods are devoid of fiber as fiber is found only in plant foods; and it is vitally important because it binds with harmful substances in the digestive system and helps carry them away from the body so they will not have the potential to harm us. Without fiber, we may become constipated and irritable. Although many people reach for fiber in a bottle or a can, it's best consumed as whole foods such as fruits and vegetables. Fiber also helps us to feel full, which is very helpful if we're striving to maintain our weight or lose unwanted pounds.

There's been a recent growing trend toward diets that promote high protein and low carbohydrate intake. As more people become disillusioned when these high animal consumption advocating systems fail to produce permanent results, these fads will pass; especially when the consequences of their advice are proven to be dangerous in the long run.

Chapter 6

Are You Fueling Yourself or Fooling Yourself?

If we took a newspaper, crumbled it up into twenty balls and ate it, and then gulped it all down with a gallon of water, we'd feel stuffed beyond comfort. Yet, we would have obtained no significant nutrients. Similarly, just because we eat and feel full afterwards does not mean that we are well nourished. At worse, the wrong type of foods can have grave consequences on our health and wellbeing.

That's why a natural progression on the journey to self empowerment includes taking greater responsibility and control of our health. The efforts we invest in our food choices today will become the fruits of wellbeing that we will benefit from tomorrow. That's why one of the fastest ways to empower ourselves is to improve our diet.

We all recognize the immense power of food on some deep level, with its ability to lift us up and make us strong or take us down and make us weak. In distant times, food was thought to be medicine because people recognized it's ability to create health and vibrancy or cause disease and disharmony. Centuries before antibiotics and drugs were invented, natural healers, doctors, and shamans treated injuries and illness with natural plants and foods. The closest pharmacy was the garden or forest. They quickly learned which plants healed and which were poisonous because life depended on it. Today, some of the drugs that we use are derived from plants because many contain powerful active substances that have tremendous healing properties.

Along with the obvious reasons of enjoying a pain-free body, a longer lifespan, and a fitter appearance, we want to take charge of our health because a strong body and mind allow us to execute our skills more effectively in a self defense situation. Imagine having weak bones from faulty dietary habits; the chances of breaking a bone if you fall or strike your hand during a confrontation will naturally increase. But if your body is strong and resilient, the likelihood of injury–along with disease risk–decrease.

Remember, what you eat becomes a part of you; it will either assist you or weaken you. If you imagine your body as a fortress that guards your spirit, you'd want that fortress to be reinforced and fortified. Knowing that certain ingested ingredients harm your structure should cause you to think twice about your choices. When you fill up on empty junk food calories, processed sugar, white flour, and animal products, you're are not fueling your body properly. When your body is starving for fiber and nutrients, it may rebel by keeping the hunger signal on long after you have eaten. This can start a vicious cycle of willpower and self-control conflicts that encourage overeating, which may lead to unnecessary weight.

We all have to eat several times every day out of necessity, so why not turn those times into opportunities to increase our strength, vitality, and self esteem? When you choose to ingest health-promoting foods, they become the building blocks that help your body to function better physically, mentally, and emotionally. As you've discovered in the previous chapter: the fitness and diet industries don't have your best interests at heart, so isn't it time to start taking control of your own health destiny?

There is a parallel between your diet and your life; eating well means you care about yourself. When you eat something wholesome and nutritious, you affirm that you love and value your body and its needs. When you avoid foods that are disempowering, you assert that you will not tolerate junk in your body, similar to not allowing someone to abuse or negatively infringe on your psyche.

The reason there seems to be so much confusion about what we should be eating is because we've gotten further removed from our natural state. Many of today's "foods" are created in laboratories and are simply not fit for human consumption. Instead, these makeshift edibles fuel emotional problems, cognitive decline, and dietary related diseases, fanning the flames of these maladies into raging fires of health destruction.

Our body has trillions of cells that require the proper amount of nutrients to work optimally and keep us healthy. Unfortunately, many individuals today look at food more as a source of stimulation and medication, i.e. "escape," than for sustenance. A good majority of the processed products that people eat are no longer even food in the better sense of the word, but rather, fractionated, refined, and adulterated substances that exude drug-like effects on the body and mind. In the coming sections, you'll learn some of the reasons such disempowering "foods" have the power to hypnotize you to such a large extent, and find real solutions that get you back on the road to empowered health.

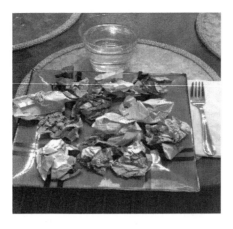

If we took a newspaper, crumbled it up into twenty balls and ate it, and then gulped it all down with a gallon of water, we'd feel stuffed beyond comfort. Yet, we would have obtained no significant nutrients.

Reclaiming Our Taste-buds and Brain Chemistry

In the not-so-distant past, we counted on our taste-buds to let us know what foods were safe to eat in the wild and what foods we should avoid. Ingesting the wrong foods in nature often meant illness or worse, while eating the right foods meant health and vitality, so our sense of taste served an important purpose: it helped us determine the foods we should consume and those we should stay away from.

Today, crafty food manufacturers have expertly hijacked our taste buds and monopolized them for their financial benefit. Along with honing the techniques of prolonging food spoilage, they mastered the pinnacle of salesmanship by perfecting the methods that make us addicted to their offerings. With extensive monetary resources at their disposal, they combined food-science with biochemistry, employing countless experts in the field to diligently study and perfect the cheapest ways to "fool" our taste buds into consuming whatever they decided to serve us. Since they gained a deep understanding of how our body works, they also learned how to exploit our natural preferences for sweet, salty, and fatty foods, along with excitatory substances seldom found in nature in large quantities.

"Craving experts" were hired to create hyperpalatable junk foods that helped trigger addictive reward pathways in our brain to maintain a steely grip of influence over our body, mind, and wallet. Product manufactures fully understood that when they refined wholesome foods—removing their water, fiber, and nutrients—and added dangerous oils, sweeteners, salt, and artificial flavors and colors—they exaggerated, suppressed, and altered the new "foods" flavors and chemical structures to elicit an enticing "mouth feel." This kept us addicted to their products.

How many of us have developed a "hyper palate" because we've been eating degraded, chemically modified, and unnaturally seasoned edibles from childhood to the present day? That simply means that our taste buds keep looking for the familiar chemical enhancers that they've always found in processed foods, which make whole foods taste mild by comparison. It's like being on a roller-coaster moving at high speeds, and immediately after, going for a ride on the lazy river—it feels as if we're hardly moving anymore. That's one of the reasons whole foods don't taste as flavorful to some people as processed foods; their taste sensitivity has decreased from being continually bombarded, numbed, and overstimulated by chemically modified foods. Chemically tweaked foods hijack the pleasure centers in our brain so that we no longer feel satisfied with the whole, unadulterated foods found in nature; our brain gets a bigger "thrill" from the roller-coaster ride of modified foods.

Today's big food conglomerates have selectively engineered foods to be like drugs;[1] once we get a taste of their edibles, our brain goes haywire and we start on the road to dependency. These habit-forming foods wreak havoc on our brain and body. We're enticed to buy short term "happiness" as sugary donuts, salty chips, and gooey desserts, but we're never told about the long term repercussions associated with dietary related diseases such as heart disease, diabetes, obesity, Attention Deficit Disorder, hyperactivity, and depression. By taking advantage of our primal drives, food manufacturers distorted our natural reactions and turned them against us. We became like just another addict who's willing to compromise her health for whatever the processed food manufacturers happen to be offering.

Because educating us about the real dangers inherent in engineered food products would be counterproductive to the financial bottom-line of processed food companies, we're essentially left at the mercy of their concoctions, which seduce both our taste-buds and brain chemistry in predictable ways.

We're not told that most processed foods are missing a very important component to our health: fiber. In the old days, they used to call it "roughage." Fiber regulates bowel activity and it helps us get rid of wastes that are harmful to our body. Think of fiber as the substance that can clean up a chemical spill. If we don't eat enough fiber, what's going to attach to the toxins? Instead, when fiber is missing, the toxins can get reabsorbed back into our blood stream.

The good news is that reclaiming our taste-buds and brain chemistry is easier than we think. The goal is to choose foods that grow from the earth—foods that are fresh —not processed or laden with sugar, salt, and a multitude of artificial flavorings, colorings, and preservatives. Our meal choices should be based on foods that are fresh, organic, and unprocessed.

The healthy carbohydrates found in fruits, veggies, beans, and grains are different from those found in most processed foods. The later cause the body's blood glucose levels to spike, while the former—sometimes referred to as complex carbohydrates—are much healthier because they don't cause the same glucose spike. If, for example, we throw a piece of paper into a fire—Poof!—it's burned very fast and is quickly gone. On the other hand, if we throw a few wood logs on a fire, we get a sustained release of energy that burns steadily for a much longer time.

The coming sections will outline the basics of good nutrition in a whole new, more empowering light.

Water-Rich or Water-Poor?

One of the repercussions of eating processed foods is dehydration; a condition that can affect our mood, appetite, and performance. It's easy to mistake thirst signals for hunger signals. When we're dehydrated, adequate blood cannot reach the brain or muscles, leaving us sleepy and lethargic. Unfortunately, many of us are sub-clinically dehydrated, which means that we're not providing adequate quantities of water to our body.

The typical Standard American Diet (S.A.D.) includes plenty of packaged, puffed, and altered foods; edibles that don't contain water and induce dehydration. If you put carrots, celery, and kale into a juicer, you'd get a fresh tasty vegetable juice. However, if you put a package of cereal or a box of diet powder mix into a juicer, you certainly would not get "cereal juice" or "diet powder juice" because these processed foods contain very little or no water.

Water serves many critical functions essential to vibrant health. It carries nutrients throughout the body while whisking the harmful waste products away from the cells; it regulates body temperature, and it maintains a healthy circulatory system. When we're dehydrated, the blood has a tendency to become thick. The consistency can start to resemble slow moving molasses rather than fast-flowing cranberry juice, which places a strain on the body's ability to deliver nutrients and oxygen to tissues. Since red blood cells carry oxygen, if their job is impeded, we can start to feel exhausted.

Our water requirements can vary, especially if we add additional water-demanding sources such as exercise, diuretics, dry environments, and certain medications to the list. That's why the body may be continually craving water.

You don't necessarily have to drink water all day long, you just need to make sure that you focus your meals around high-water content foods. The two categories of foods with the highest water content are fresh fruits and vegetables. This is one of the reasons you want a good portion of your diet to be abundant in water-rich foods–to make sure that you're properly hydrated.

If you enjoy drinking clean water, one of the best ways to enhance the taste experience and add an abundance of antioxidants to the liquid is by including herbal teas such a hibiscus, rooibos, dandelion, or chamomile. Additionally, a small amount of pure blueberry, cranberry, or pomegranate juice can be added to clean water to make a diluted juice. Incorporating high-antioxidant pure juices in small amounts slightly sweetens the water, encouraging us to drink more volume. This is one of the fastest way of adding antioxidants to our liquids. Green powders are also helpful and can be mixed with water and carried for sipping throughout the day.

The more whole, unprocessed foods you incorporate into your meals, the less chance of dehydration. High-water content foods such as fruits and vegetables ensure that there is less room for less desirable processed foods, which tend to "suck" the water out of your system. Processed foods and animal products may accelerate premature aging, both in the brain and the body. Animal products are loaded with cholesterol and saturated fat and don't have a speck of fiber. They lack the phytonutrients we desperately need for exceptional health and wellbeing.

The phytonutrients and antioxidant's found in whole foods help you stay strong and energetic—increasing every attribute you need to protect and defend yourself. If we cut an apple in half, the exposed surfaces will start to turn brown or oxidize. However, if we squeeze some fresh lemon juice on the exposed surfaces, the progression of oxidation is greatly diminished because the ascorbic acid (vitamin C) and other phytonutrients inherent in the lemon juice act as antioxidants, preserving the apple tissue longer.

Being strong and empowered means you start to get control of what you put into your body. When you choose whole foods that grow from the earth, you fuel yourself with real foods instead of fooling yourself with depleting and disease-promoting makeshift edibles. Science-based evidence supports the position that minimally processed, whole plant foods provide the most optimal nutritional foundation. We benefit by getting the macronutrients in the right quantities and increased micronutrients.

A diet based on plant matter is also generally lower in fat. The other benefits are what you are *not* eating:

cholesterol, saturated fat, hormones, antibiotics, and pesticides. You also get plenty of fiber which is critical for removing toxins from your system, and lowering blood sugar and cholesterol. When you eat foods according to these principles, you become stronger, healthier, and more balanced.

Putting Food to the Empowerment Test

One of the best ways to test a food for wholesome integrity is by asking questions. Just as we can cultivate higher standards in our relationships to build our self esteem and life satisfaction, food should also pass our high demands for its nutritional content. That means we obviously want to avoid foods that are disempowering—those that steal our vibrancy and health, along with those that may seduce us with empty (calories) promises. The goal is to go for real foods that empower us with positive, long-lasting physical, mental, and emotional effects.

It's often useful to put food to your own empowerment test. This can be a series of questions that you choose to ask yourself before you decide if you wish to eat a particular food. They may include the following, along with your own unique questions:

- **Is this food found this way in nature?** If you take frozen berries out of a bag, they still look relatively the same as if you picked them fresh once they defrosted. However, if you take a cookie from a box, can you find it in that state in nature? If the answer is no, it's a good indication that it's a processed food that may be disempowering to you in the long run.

- **Is this food rich in phytonutrients?** When foods are whole and unadulterated they contain substantial amounts of empowering nutrients. An organic apple is filled with many phytonutrients, along with many other whole foods. Most salty chips, however, are not. Considering whether the food that you're thinking of ingesting is rich in phytonutrients can help you focus on more quality choices rather than nutrient depleting ones.

- **Is this food rich in fiber?** Whole plant foods are loaded with fiber, a critical substance for our wellbeing. Processed foods have very little fiber, if at all, robbing you of this crucial material. A pear would be loaded with fiber, but a steak would not a have speck.

- **Is this food rich in water?** Fruits and vegetables are loaded with water—they're water-rich. Whole grains and beans will not contain water before cooking, but will absorb substantial amounts of water during the cooking process. Even though whole grains and beans do not contain the high water content of fruits and vegetables, they still provide nutrients, fiber, and much goodness.

- **Does this food have "stuff" I don't want?** Whole, fresh fruits and vegetables will not have anything added. They usually come right from the farm to the grocer. Comparatively, most processed foods have "stuff" added that's disempowering including sugar, salt, oil, artificial flavors and colors, and hard-to-pronounce ingredients that sometimes require a pharmaceutical dictionary to define

–definitely not what you're looking for in empowered nutrition.

- **Is this food addicting for me?** Whole foods that grow from the earth are rarely addicting unless they're tampered with mechanically. If the food you're considering cannot pass this question, chances are great that it shouldn't be on your menu. As you now know, most foods that have been modified are addicting. If you're continually thinking about the same types of foods, chances are very great that they are addicting for you.

- **Will this food empower or disempower my body and mind?** If you want more empowerment ask yourself this question before you start eating. Know that processed foods and animal products take away from your empowerment, leading you on the road to poor health, accelerated aging, and weight-gain. In contrast, empowering foods give you qualities that support your health, cognitive function, and add to your youthful-glow. Chose to love yourself with empowering foods.

Your Empowerment Team: Wholesome Foods

Whole foods are those that add nutrition and health-value to your mind and body. They provide much needed vitamins, minerals, and macro and micro nutrients and work hard to protect you from harmful diseases. They're foods that add to your empowerment, making you stronger and more resilient.

Building a happy relationship with food starts with awareness and discernment. Awareness of what healthy foods are and making the conscious and deliberate choice to consume them. Take a look at the following partial list of empowering foods and consider implementing them into your healthy lifestyle.

Greens—There are a wide variety of greens to chose from and all are loaded with impressive amounts of antioxidants, fiber, and distinct flavors. Think of greens as a starting point for your colorful salad or an important addition to any dish. Discover kale, collard greens, red or green leaf lettuce, spinach, Swiss chard, bok choy, endive, dandelion, radicchio, watercress, arugula, parsley, and explore greens you've never tried before. Consider including greens in your smoothies to increase your intake.

Vegetables—There are countless varieties of vegetables, which give salads and most dishes enticing flavors and textures. The secret with vegetables is to rotate them often; this gives you a wider variety of nutrients and helps make sure that you're getting the antioxidants that you need. Vegetables are extremely versatile, and can be enjoyed in salads, soups, side dishes, main courses, or just for snacking with a healthy dip like hummus. Consider artichokes, asparagus, bell peppers (red, yellow, orange, green), broccoli, Brussels sprouts, cabbage, cauliflower, celery, leeks, onions, sprouts (variety), and much more.

Starchy Vegetables—Starchy vegetables add satiety and complex carbohydrates to a salad or any meal. Consider pumpkin, purple potatoes, radishes, sweet potatoes, summer Squash (zucchini), yams, and much more. One technique to save time during a busy workweek is to steam starchy vegetables on the weekend and store them in glass containers in the refrigerator. They can be quickly reheated and tossed on top of any salad, or added to soups and other dishes.

Fruits and Berries—Think of fruits and berries as your dessert—like natures candy. They're bursting with sweetness, fiber, antioxidants, vitamins, and minerals. The secret with fruit is to have a wide variety, especially fruit salads, so every time you open the refrigerator, you see a luscious cornucopia of fruits in the fridge. Focus on pomegranates, mangos, strawberries, kiwis, pineapples, apricots, blackberries, blueberries, boysenberries, cantaloupe, cherries, papaya, pears, and more. When fresh fruit is not in season, consider storing frozen fruits and berries to use in smoothies, oatmeal, or as an addition to cultured coconut milk (So Delicious brand).

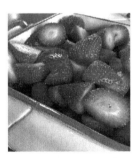

Think of fruits and berries as your dessert—like natures candy.

Legumes—Legumes include beans, peas, and lentils. They're a wonderful source of protein and fiber and satisfy the appetite because of their slow release of complex carbohydrates. Cook legumes ahead of time and store them in the refrigerator or the freezer to add to soups, dressings, main dishes, or salads. Invite black beans, garbanzo beans, lentils, peas, red beans, tempeh, tofu, and pinto beans into your meals.

Whole Grains—Grains are good sources of complex carbohydrates, fiber, and nutrients. They can be cooked ahead of time and stored in the refrigerator for later use. Add grains to salads, as an addition to any vegetables, and to soups. Many have a delightfully nutty flavor and texture. Consider amaranth, brown rice, millet, oatmeal, quinoa, and wild rice.

Nuts and Seeds—High in protein, fiber, and healthy fats, these concentrated dynamos should be eaten raw, unsalted, and in moderation. Be sure to chew nuts and seeds well, until they reach a liquid consistency for better absorption. Sprinkle a few on your salads or incorporate them into your smoothie. Consider almonds, Brazil nuts, chia seeds, hemp seeds, Sacha Inchi seeds, pine nuts, walnuts, and flaxseeds.

Fresh Herbs—Chopped fresh herbs add distinctive flavor and additional nutrients to any salad or dish. Consider dill, mint, chives, basil, garlic, cilantro, tarragon, thyme, oregano, and marjoram. Dried herbs and spices add a powerful antioxidant boost to any meal, so experiment with adding Ceylon cinnamon to your oatmeal or smoothie, rosemary to soups or potatoes, and toss a few leaves of basil to your clean drinking water for added flavor.

Focus on Adding in the Good

Chances are great that you're attached to your favorite
foods. If someone told you to stop eating a food that you've
been eating for decades, you'd probably get defensive.
That's very common—even if you know that it's not in your
best health interest. Many of us have emotional bonds with
our favorite foods. Gooey, fatty sauces may bring back
memories of happy family dinners, festive parties, and
special occasions.

It's easy to keep yourself from improving when you
know you're capable of so much more because change is
often considered risky. You may fear losing the acceptance
of people you depend on who may not like the new
direction that you're going; your new and more
empowering food ideas can seem odd and intimidating to
others. So it becomes a multifaceted challenge to avoid less
than healthy foods.

You may want to stay with your less-than-perfect
food choices out of habit, addiction, or emotional ties, and
may not want anyone to take them away from you,
regardless of the reasons. You may recall that as a child,
anything "off-limits" meant that it was somehow "good" or
something that simply had to be "tried" when the
opportunity presented itself. So when someone restricts you
in some way, you may rebel, often unconsciously. And even
if you didn't want the items in the past, their prohibition
may, at the very least, pique your interest and curiosity.

That's why the "taking away" strategy often fails,
because many people rebel against having to give
something up. A far more effective plan is to add more of
what you want to your meals. One empowering idea that

can increase your chance of success is the "Good, Better, Best," philosophy described in *The Pillars of Health* (Pierre 2013). It's a philosophy based on continual improvement. You start by being kinder to yourself by putting in good foods, good thoughts, good ideas, and surrounding yourself with good and kind people. *The more good you put in, the less room remains for less desirable options.*

This frame of mind takes the pressure off being perfect. It keeps you focused simply on looking for better options. The idea is to always try to improve what you're eating. There should never be any blame or guilt involved because the focus is on doing better. There are no such things as "bad" foods. Labeling foods as "bad," "off-limits," and "undesirable," simply leads to their mystique, which further fuels our desire.

It makes sense to simply add more of what you want into your meals. The more good, wholesome plant foods you keep adding, the less room remains on your plate –and in your stomach–for less desirable ones.

All of us have developed eating habits that are not in our best health interests and it's easier to let certain foods fade away from our life than others. It seems like one day we take two steps forward and then next day we take one step back. That's just fine as long as we keep focused on the direction we want to go.

Change can test your internal resources and your determination, especially when you start to transition away from habit-forming foods. If you're not used to eating plants, simply going out of your way to include a vegetable in your meal may be a big deal for you. That's fine. We all have to start somewhere and you can only start from exactly where you are. The secret is to add in as much good as possible.

Tips to Add In More Wholesome Foods

- Make a shopping list before you go to the grocery store to avoid temptation. Focus on adding more fresh, nutrient-bursting wholesome foods to your cart. These are the foods that will end up in your refrigerator, pantry, and, eventually, in your stomach. The foods you chose to eat will eventually become a part of your body and mind.

- Buy whole grains and beans in bulk to save money, and reduce packaging and waste. Grains and beans can last for years if stored in a cool and dry place, making them great investments against increasing food costs. Whole grains are usually much cheaper compared to processed foods which tend to be both wallet-depleting and health-destroying.

- Invest in glass storage containers of all sizes. Refrigerate or freeze cooked grains and chopped vegetables; and pre-make your next day's meal to store in a glass container in the fridge to take to work.

- If you're used to eating dessert after your meal, try adding fruit. The sweetness and fiber helps to satisfy most cravings for sweets.

- Add more vegetables and greens to every meal and eat these first before anything else. When you fill up on nutrient-dense foods first, you leave less room in the stomach for less desirable offerings.

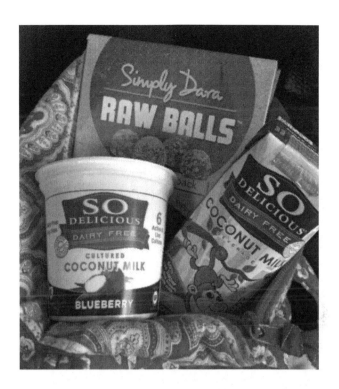

Keep healthy snacks in your purse and a small cooler in your car. Good choices include fresh fruit, raw nuts, raw seeds, chopped vegetables, and organic food bars such as the Organic Food Bars, Evo Hemp, Boku Bars, and the 22 Day brands; along with Simply Dara Raw Balls. Your car cooler can keep items that need to be refrigerated for short times, including cultured coconut milk (So Delicious brand), almond milk and coconut milk (So Delicious brand), and other travel items to take on the road for healthy eating.

- Make a collage of your favorite fruits and vegetables and place it on your fridge. Looking at the cornucopia of nutrient-bursting, colorful whole foods may inspire you to make better and healthier choices.

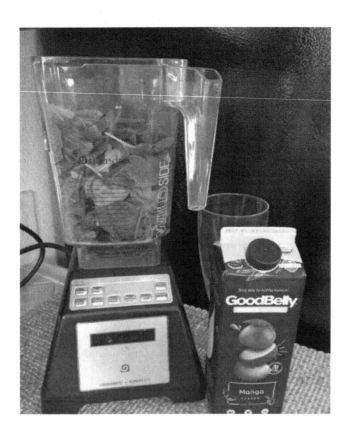

Sneak more greens into your day by blending them with your favorite nut milk, juice, or clean water. Your green drink can travel with you in a glass or stainless steel container for sipping throughout the day.

Chapter 7

Releasing an Abusive Food-Affair

All pleasurable experiences hold the potential to become addictions. Thrilling adventures don't surround us 24 hours per day, but "entertainment food" does; through magazines, commercials, billboards, fast food offerings, and enticing packages available everywhere we turn. Since we must eat several times each day out of necessity, it becomes easy and tempting to succumb to feasting on denatured foods because they're constantly in our face and often the cheapest (financially in the short term) option available.

An abusive food-affair can start at any time, especially when we lose our connection with ourselves. If we hardly spend time on introspection or building a spiritual connection to the earth, and most of our time is spent on activities that are focused "outside" of ourselves, it may be easier to turn to stimulating entertainment that gives our brain a temporary "high," because we're in a constant state of "low."

When the processed food industry altered whole foods, they found a way to override our willpower by tricking our brain and body to create cravings; ensuring rampant dependency on their products. Many people blame themselves for food addictions because no one explains the sneaky, lab-created reasons behind their infatuations with sugary cookies, gooey pies, greasy pizza, and creamy ice cream; the food companies are certainly not going to disclose that information and act against their own financial self-interests. So when we're depressed or angry we often don't reach for a green leafy salad or fresh broccoli but instead go for processed foods because they provide our brain with the biggest "high." It's almost impossible to use whole, unprocessed foods as medication because they don't provide the same "high" as modified edibles.

Like predatory charlatans, most processed foods seduce our taste buds and body chemistry by lighting up the pleasure centers in our brain. If we try to quit, the temporary repercussions are often nausea, irritability, headaches, shakiness, lethargy, insomnia, and vicious cravings—defining symptoms of withdrawal from an addictive substance. Because processed foods laden with fat, sugar, and salt activate dopamine receptors in the brain, we seek more of them to attain the same "high" that will generate the same amount of pleasure. Unfortunately, these "foods" cause a *temporary* high that's often followed by a crash, leading to a cycle of food abuse.

Many individuals are using processed foods as a substitute for love, affection, validation, and meaningful human contact. Some overeat to numb themselves. Processed foods becomes the "intermediary" that *temporarily* alleviates the emotions of boredom, grief, depression, emptiness, loneliness, and rejection.

A food addiction seems to satisfy some momentary needs—but not for long. Since processed foods can't fill the void adequately, the true emptiness never goes away and we're left wanting more. One of the most damaging things about an abusive food affair is that it keeps us from getting in touch with and learning to satisfy our true needs and desires.

Abusing the body by binging, purging, and obsessing about processed foods (and it's usually processed foods—really, who has an obsession with cabbage, lettuce, bell peppers, or kale?) is something that people often keep to themselves—similar to keeping an abusive relationship with a spouse secret—because they're too embarrassed and ashamed to tell others. Often, family and friends don't have a clue that their loved one is binging or purging in seclusion. Many people who are addicted to food have repeated their addictive food patterns so many times that they eventually just "go through the motions" automatically without even thinking about it. Some restrict their food intake because the self-inflicted deprivation provides them with a sense of comfort and control. Regardless of the many ways food can be abused—it's always self-abuse.

Food addictions have both physical and emotional components. They self-sabotage inner peace and add to our self-destruction. Physically addicting foods, which are often loaded with processed sugar, spike our "feel good" brain chemicals, but often cause their depletion in the long run. The natural brain receptors for dopamine, after continuous processed food bombardment, depletes our stores of serotonin, which diminishes our sense of wellbeing. This makes us even more vulnerable to depression and serious cravings between our "fixes."

Dealing with emotions that trigger food binges or purges is very important. Some feelings masquerade as biochemical influences from processed foods, which often contain excitotoxins such as aspartame (commonly found in sodas). Certain additives can trigger allergic reactions, headaches, and long-term neurological problems. The sulfites found in wines and some restaurant foods may also trigger reactions in sensitive people.

Any abusive habit may temporarily help us to avoid the pain of not having our real needs met. Unaddressed and untreated food addictions are a guaranteed way to sabotage any real possibility of true health and emotional peace. The addiction becomes an attempt to unconsciously fill the emptiness we feel inside, which can only be filled with a connection to ourselves.

There are a number of strategies that can assist with releasing an abusive food affair. The first, and most important, is to shift the diet towards whole foods, adding in fresh, unprocessed foods in increasing quantities to meals so less or no room remains for processed ones.

The goal is to make eating whole foods a *lifestyle habit*, which allows you to eat without restriction; gaining essential nutrients, lasting vibrancy, and abundant health. It also cuts the strings of processed food manufacturers control, allowing you to reclaim your power and get in tune with your real nutritional needs. The concepts introduced in this book strive to inspire self-loving choices that put you in charge of facing and embracing your emotional needs. Once you acknowledge, release, and heal an abusive food affair, you'll create an empowered state of freedom for yourself, and help others do the same.

Helpful Tips

- Increase the amount of fresh whole foods in your meals. Begin a meal with whole foods, leaving anything else for after.

- Surround yourself by a supportive environment and include books or DVD's that help you stay on track. Consider *The 30 Day Unprocessed Challenge* by Chef AJ and John Pierre to help you incorporate more whole foods into your day; along with *Ultimate Weight Loss* by Chef AJ and John Pierre.

- Look for emotional triggers. Self-sabotaging behaviors often begin as traumatic events. Abusive food-affairs are often attempts to deal with difficult-to-handle emotional issues. Consider keeping a journal to help process your emotions.

- Donate your scale. Focus on how you feel and function and how your clothes fit. Don't let a number dictate your worthiness or self esteem.

- Use alone-time to tune-in to yourself instead of tuning-out with food.

- Don't try to use food as an escape; instead, contemplate. Spend quality time with yourself, even if it's only for a few extra minutes during the day. Focus those moments on self reflection and getting in touch with your inner voice.

- Don't be afraid to seek professional help. Consider reaching out to others who have experience and success with eating disorders for additional support and assistance.

Cheese Addiction: No Laughing Matter

Many people claim they have a harder time giving up cheese than cigarettes. That's by manufactured design, of course.

Cheese and it's byproducts are routinely found in most processed packaged foods, including frozen dinners. In an excellent book titled *Breaking the Food Seduction*, Dr. Neal Barnard discusses how casein breaks down during digestion to produce casomorphins which are thought to contribute to the mother-infant bond that occurs during nursing. A cup of milk contains six grams of casein but it is especially concentrated in cheese which is why it's theorized that pizza is one of American's favorite foods. If we were to take away the cheese from all pizzas, most people would not be attracted to eating them.

The goal is to break out of the addiction and embrace the non-addictive nature of whole, plant based foods. These foods are not drugs and they will not lead us astray. Real whole foods can improve health, peace of mind, and assist with the sustainability of our planet. Let these be the overriding factors that inspire you to open your wallet when you shop for food.

Your Friendly Food Diary

Just as a lack of awareness can be an adversary in self defense situations, a lack of insight can also become a hindrance when you try to get healthy, shed some unwanted body fat, or heal a food addiction. That's why keeping a food diary is a powerful way to raise your nutritional self awareness.

It's common to lose track of what's eaten during a busy day, and a food diary can allow you to focus on what, where, when, and why you eat, helping you to recognize any eating patterns. Writing in a food diary puts you in greater control and allows you to reflect on your thoughts and feelings. Since it's often easy to miss the connection between the food you eat and your moods, noting the pattern can help you make different and more empowering choices ahead of time. It allows you to take responsibility, building your confidence and power.

The goal is to write down what you're eating and how you feel while eating. There's no need to measure every gram of food fanatically; that's often counterproductive and not necessary. If you ate a candy bar at work because you felt famished and that was the only thing available, you can decide to bring something healthy to have on hand the very next day. Your food diary should help you feel more accountable and give you renewed motivation and encouragement. Increased awareness also helps release stress.

Take a look at the following suggestions and pointers about keeping a food diary.

Food Diary Tips

- **Check for meal patterns:** If you skip meals frequently and allow too much time to lapse between eating, you may be setting yourself up to overeat later. Experiment with adding healthy snacks to decrease the time lapse between meals. Note the results in your food diary. Many individuals believe that it's fine to skip meals and then end up splurging later, but that's often taxing on the digestive system and may lead to binging. Also note if you're eating more when you watch television or when you're out with friends (or certain people). This can be an unconscious habit or a way of dealing with nervousness or boredom. Your food diary will help illuminate these patterns, giving you an opportunity to change your actions if they're disempowering.

- **Look for triggers:** Become conscious of the effect your moods have on your eating. We often eat when we're bored or depressed. Sometimes just seeing a picture of food or smelling it can increase cravings and ignite an ingrained habit of eating. Look for triggers in your food diary to help you recognize and change behaviors. If you notice that you eat during the evening only while watching television, it may be helpful to turn it off. Eating crunchy foods such as chips are often craved during times of stress since chomping on harder foods helps to release tension in the jaw, a common place where we hold stress. Try substituting healthier crunchy vegetables for processed chips if crunching helps you release tension. Other stress-relieving techniques include deep breathing, a quick walk, stretching, or foam-rolling tense muscles. Eating junk food during stressful times only adds-on unwanted pounds and helps create dietary-related diseases, leading to additional stress and guilt.

- **Have a plan:** A food diary illuminates the triggers and patterns that may lead to overeating and makes them very obvious. Once you recognize the antagonistic triggers and patters that are holding you back, you can formulate a plan. The plan can include ways of interrupting the patterns or avoiding the triggers until they no longer have any power over you. If you always feel tempted when you pass a bakery on your way home, see if you can chose a slightly different route (if it's safe). If you notice that most of your emotional eating happens between dinner and bedtime, interrupt the pattern by brushing your teeth immediately after dinner. Try scheduling a different relaxing activity such as an aromatherapy foot soak, deep breathing, visualization, yoga, stretching, or reviewing some of the fitness drills shown in later chapters. The key is to break the patterns that are health-depleting and build new habits that are empowering.

- **Keep your food diary handy:** It's easy to forget writing down what you eat, and certain foods such as candy and salty snacks tend to get forgotten. However, everything you eat adds up, both in calorie-load and nutrients. That's why keeping your food diary close and handy is important; to jot down meals, snacks, and that "little bite" of something. If writing everything down feels like a chore, try it for only a few weeks to uncover some patterns and triggers. See if it's helpful and feel free to come back to your food diary at any time.

- **Listen to hunger signals:** It's important to get in tune with your appetite. We often eat simply because the clock says so even if we're not hungry and deprive ourselves of nourishment because we feel it's not the "right" time to eat. However, when you listen to your body and its needs, you start to eat when you feel the need and become more sensitive to what you intuitively feel drawn to. The fuller you feel, the less you generally enjoy the food. The more hungry you feel, the more you enjoy eating. They key is to eat at when you feel hungry enough to where you feel satisfied afterwards.

- **Eat with awareness:** We're often on automatic pilot when it comes to eating. Practice conscious eating by relaxing and eating mindfully in a calm environment. Clear the table of clutter, shut off the television, put on soft classical music, and make your food look appealing on your plate. If you're eating in someone else's company, try to keep the conversation pleasant. Prepare yourself wholesome fresh meals and share them with family and friends.

Part III

Be Your Own Bodyguard

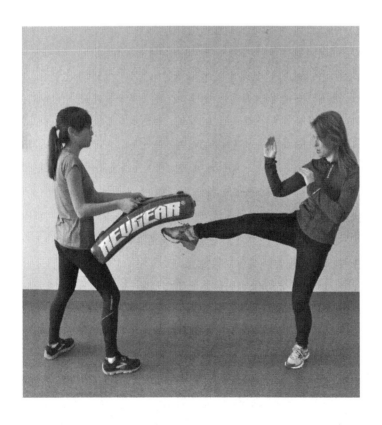

Chapter 8

Prepared Resistance

We often think that violence happens to other people, but not us. It's certainly difficult and unpleasant to visualize a crazed criminal trying to break into our home because it brings up feelings of panic, terror, and helplessness. The stuff of our worst nightmares are often thoughts of a personal assault or our loved ones being harmed, so it's far easier to push these uncomfortable thoughts and feelings aside and dive deeper into our comfortable blankets of denial; consoling ourselves with the notion that law enforcement or our spouse, neighbor, cat, or the tooth-fairy will come to our aid in time to protect us and our children from harm.

Unfortunately in today's world, it's more than just naive to believe that the police—or anyone else for that matter—will arrive just in time to help you during a dangerous situation—it's downright dangerous and potentially lethal. There are countless scenarios where you may not be able to call law enforcement because of the lack of reception, a dead battery, or a lost, stolen, or broken cell phone. In some cases, it may come as an unpleasant surprise to learn that no one is available to help you in your greatest time of danger.

This is exactly what happened to an Oregon woman recently when she called 911 to report than an aggressor was trying to break into her house. She was told by the dispatcher that no one was available to come to her aid due to budget cuts. Imagine the horror of hearing the following sentence as a vicious attacker is breaking into *your* home: "Uh, I don't have anybody to send out there. You know, obviously, if he comes inside the residence and assaults you, can you ask him to go away?"[1] Tragically, the man broke into the house and the woman was choked and sexually assaulted.

There are instances where, even when law enforcement arrived quickly, it was still too late; and, while it's important to alert the police immediately (if you can without putting yourself in greater danger) in a given emergency to ask for assistance, it's hardly realistic to assume that they'll magically appear on your doorstep in seconds to stop an attacker who just broke into your house. So fully counting on *anyone* to come to your aid and save you and your family during a life-threatening situation may be a strategy that you may want to reconsider. The goal of this book is to help you foster a *survival mind set*, which includes taking responsibility for your personal safety; the goal is for you to *be your own bodyguard.*

When you cultivate effective skills and an empowered mindset, you boost your self confidence and self esteem. You metaphorically take yourself from being a passive passenger in life to an active driver who's fully in charge of where you want to go. You take back your power and authority to take care of yourself, and you do so to the best of your ability. The aim of this book is to help you increase that ability.

When you practice and train mentally and physically (and help others to do the same) you take greater control of your personal destiny and assist others to gain greater control of theirs. Empowering yourself not only helps you–it helps everyone. If an assailant tries to break into your home, would you rather have people around you with effective training and a survival mindset or would you prefer to be surrounded by panicked and helpless individuals who didn't have a clue about what to do? That's why you want to empower both yourself and everyone around you–empowerment benefits everyone.

Prepared Resistance

As adults, most of us prepare for something almost every day in some shape or form. We prepare water and snacks to take with us on a long hike, knowing that without them we'll experience the discomfort of thirst and hunger. We prepare flashlights and blankets for the possibility of losing electricity when a storm is coming our way because we want to avoid being cold and in the dark. We even prepare for an important meeting or job interview because we know that prepping ahead of time will help insure our success. There are countless examples of how we prepare all the time without even giving it much thought simply because it's the common sense and practical thing to do.

Oddly, when the topic of self protection comes up, words like "paranoid," "suspicious," and "insecure" often come up. It seems that taking a proactive approach to the most important and valuable thing that we have–our life and the lives of our loved ones–is not currently trendy or fashionable. There's no glitz, glamour, or entertainment value attached to the subject.

Prepared resistance is all about making yourself ready to deal with a potentially dangerous confrontation which is not initiated by you. The focus is on strengthening your attributes, which means making yourself stronger –both mentally and physically, and more aware and savvy.

159

The reason that you prepare to defend yourself today is so that you'll have a better outcome at some time in the future than you would have if you didn't prepare.

Your preparation is empowering; don't let anyone else tell you otherwise. If people respond negatively (hard to believe but it happens) to your desire to learn to defend yourself, simply sit them down and have them watch a few YouTube videos that deal with real life self defense situations. Search for videos of real confrontations and see what they look like. Watch many videos—not just one—to get a broader perspective. This will give everyone a better idea of just how quickly and unexpectedly violence can escalate. Ask yourself whether you'd have the time to grab something out of your bag during a situation like that. Being prepared means you live your life in reality not delusion, which is an empowering place to be.

Remember, in an assault situation, time often works against you and for the attacker because he has the element of surprise—after all, who *expects* to be assaulted? Career criminals who aggressively go after your life or property won't give you a second chance to compose yourself or get a weapon out of your purse—*there is no "time-out" in a self defense situation*. That's why your immediate reaction is crucially important.

In a robbery situation, it's best to give the robber your jewelry, money, and car keys if that's what he want's —because the goal is to escape with your life. If an aggressor is looking for your wallet or jewelry, give it up quickly by throwing it at him or away from the direction that you want to run to. A thief will go for the goods while a predator will go for you and not your valuables. At that point you will know his true intentions. However, if the aggressor is intent on harming you, one of the best ways to survive an attack (besides prevention of course) is to cause injury.

If you're not actively and aggressively injuring your attacker, then chances are great that you are the one who's getting injured. What's missing in many crime-protection programs is that they don't disclose that you must expect to be injured. Really, if fully armed and trained police officers get hurt during altercations, you have to face the same facts.

Another frequently made mistake is waiting for the "right" time to react. You try to talk yourself out of overreacting, thinking that a better time will come when you will make your move. In reality, what you really want is a "safe" time. Unfortunately, when you're in the midst of an assault situation that *safe time is over* and it's never going to get better than it is at that moment.

There's no reason for you to be embarrassed or self-conscious in getting prepared to defend yourself. It's the strong, savvy, practical, and responsible way to live.

It's More than Just About You

If you're attacked, there's a lot more at stake than just your life. The truth is that your wellbeing—or lack of—effects more than just you; it effects every person and animal that loves and cares about you. That means that if a criminal assaults you—he also attacks your loved ones, your acquaintances, and your livelihood in *countless ways.*

You see, if you've never faced a violent assault in your life, it's hard to imagine what people who have often go through as a result. Most are *never* the same. Trauma has a way of changing people, often in profound ways.

Some individuals start to sleep with a baseball bat next to their bed after surviving an attack. Others are afraid to leave the house during certain hours (or at all). An individual will sometimes go through what most people would consider extreme lengths to avoid anything that even reminds them of the attack. Each person who survives trauma deals with it in a unique way, and there's no way of knowing what those coping mechanisms will be until after the fact. The point is that violence leaves more that just physical damage, it also leaves psychological and emotional scars that can last a lifetime.

Whatever injuries you sustain during an attack (particularly if they're disabling or disfiguring) may continue to haunt both you and everyone who knows you. Since all injury is traumatic on some level, even if there are no outward signs of harm, the psychological and emotional devastation can often be far more severe and debilitating. To put it into greater perspective: your parents won't have the same daughter or son they had before the assault; your siblings won't have the same sister or brother; your children won't have the same parent; your employer won't have the same employee; your dog won't have the same companion; your friend won't have the same friend. Because *you will likely never be the same*. Often, because of the trauma that individuals experience during and after the attack (people often continue to replay the assault in their minds), everyone that cares about them also becomes traumatized to a certain extent.

An aggressor who makes a choice to assault you doesn't care how your resulting injury or trauma from his assault will effect you or others. He couldn't care less that you won't be able to drive your grandmother to the grocery store if he breaks your arm. It's not even a thought in his mind to consider how your pain and injury will effect everyone who knows and cares about you. And if an assailant takes your life then everyone suffers a loss as well. Let's face it, you—like every being—are unique and irreplaceable, so losing you becomes a loss for every loved one and individual in the future who could have been positively touched by your smile, your words of encouragement, your assistance, your company, and so much more.

So when you fight back against an assailant, you don't just fight back for yourself. You fight back for all your loved ones who want to see you happy, healthy, and whole.

Each Attack is Unique

When you're forced into an unintentional self defense scenario, you'll be under intense pressure to judge your immediate capabilities and opportunities in your unique circumstances. You'll be the only one who can make the personal decision to use physical force, become passive, or a combination of the two options at different times; and that's because each attack and assailant is different.

To be clear, there is really no right or wrong method when it comes to defending yourself. Some individuals have escaped from an attacker by pleading with and begging him into giving up on an assault; though it's hardly realistic to rely on a sudden awakening of an assailants conscience. Attackers are rarely sympathetic—if they were, they wouldn't be engaged in an assault to begin with. Other individuals have escaped to safety by tricking the assailant with their acting skills and made-up stories that may have temporarily confused and bewildered the attacker until they found an opportunity to escape to safety. Additionally, some women have feigned helplessness to drop the guard of their assailant to gain a better advantage when they finally fought back.

Years ago, a horrific serial killer who was fond of luring young men and boys to his house, solicited a young man to come to his place with him. When he tried to handcuff the young man, he managed to escape after fighting back by punching the assailant in the face. His act led to the capture of this brutal predator. The young man not only saved his own life, but possibly countless others.

Some assailants are fond of luring women into a waiting trap by feigning helplessness and weakness by wearing fake casts or sitting in a wheelchair to lower a woman's guard. They feign immobility, ask for assistance, and play on the woman's sympathy and compassion. One such brutal killer, who had been viciously assaulting and murdering women for years, began his routine by asking girls if they could help him get his sailboat on to his car while wearing a fake cast. He then grabbed them and threw them in his car. Fortunately, one woman resisted and fought for her life, even thought he pulled a gun on her to try to subdue her. As he put the gun away though, she fought again and managed to escape as he tried to handcuff her. Thankfully, because of her resistance and escape, he was eventually caught.

Understanding "Crime Scene Number 2"

Without a moral conscience and with plenty of violent intent, an assailant will use every trick in the book to gain the upper hand. That means that if he can lie to make an assault easier on himself, he definitely will. That's why any promises or requests an assailant may make, no matter how genuinely delivered, should be automatically considered as highly suspect. Deceiving others is a way of life for most criminals and they'll do anything to get what they want with the least amount of work and effort. If an aggressor promises you safety and security as a reward for your complacency and cooperation, there's a high probability that he's lying.

When an assailant says: "Come with me, I'm not going to hurt you," why would you believe him? If someone is making you do anything forcibly against your will, why would changing a location be better for you? It won't. Criminals don't threaten others just for a chance to have a pleasant conversation over a cup of tea. Remember, they see you as a "target." You're just another addition to their rap sheet if they get caught. How do you reason with a person like that? Someone who's likely so desensitized from harming a long list of others and who see's no value in you as a person other than for his personal aims.

It's common for individuals to want to believe an aggressor's false promises because we all have a tendency to impart our honorable values on others if we're genuine and honest ourselves. Unfortunately, assailants are anything but sincere. Most are criminals without a conscience who don't think twice about lying, cheating, stealing, assaulting, and killing.

Why do criminals want to take someone to a different location? Because they want isolation and control; they want to make sure that no one will see or hear what they plan on doing. That's why "crime scene number 2" must never occur. In his brilliant book, *Strong on Defense*,

Stanford Strong, who taught police and SWAT officers how to defend themselves, says the following about crime scene number 2:

...“The sole purpose in moving you is to get you out of sight and reduce the chance of intervention. You wind up isolated and at the mercy of the merciless. A crime scene #2 investigation usually involves murder, rape, sometimes sadism and torture.”

“Never allow the attacker to move you to a more isolated spot (behind the wall, over to the hedge). If he's only a robber, he doesn't need to move you. A rapist and some killers are looking for isolation, seclusion. Risk everything to stop a criminal from moving you to crime scene #2. Risk injury. Risk being shot. Lousy options now are better than no options later.” [1]

Just because an assailant transports his target to another location does not mean that death will come swiftly. Some attackers sell their targets into the sex slave industry or force them into pimping for them. And occasionally a "crime scene number 2" scenario can last for many torturous years for kidnap targets.

Recently, in Cleveland Ohio, three women were rescued after being held captive for over a decade. They were kidnapped at ages 14, 16, and 20. Upon their rescue, they described suffering prolonged sexual and psychological abuse, and forced miscarriages. Law enforcement officials stated that the women were apparently bound by ropes and chains and kept in different rooms; they were not allowed outside.[2] The outcome is always far worse at the second location.

If an assailant breaks into your home with intent to harm, your residence can quickly turn into a "crime scene number 2" location because you're already in a secluded environment where few outsiders can see or hear your struggles. You're essentially isolated, with the possibility of additional young family members present who can be used to further control you. This is one of the reasons that role-play and emergency drills are so important to practice ahead of time.

If you're accosted in a public setting and the assailant want's to transport you to another location by threatening you with a weapon, you're better off taking a risk in public than going to a secluded location with him. Take your chances and run. If you're grabbed, struggle, hit, bite, and scream. If you fear being shot or stabbed, your chances are reduced of this happening in a public setting. Remember, a criminal does not want to be seen (or worse −videotaped) and incarcerated, so there's more pressure on him to escape the prying eyes, speed-dial phones, and today's abundant smart-phone cameras. If he decides to shoot you immediately when you struggle, the chances are very high that he is a killer and would have done that in a secluded location (at his leisure), with a greater chance of making sure that he didn't miss.

Criminals understand that if they decide to shoot in a public setting, the noise alone will alert people nearby. They generally don't want to stick around for that. If he shoots at you, he can always miss or hit a non-vital area. Once he flees others can come to your aid. If he stabs you in the first few minutes of the attack, what do you think your chances would be with him in a secluded location but with more time and less pressure? The second location takes the pressure off and allows the predator to do exactly what he want's at his sadistic leisure.

Your best chance of survival may be to take the risk in a public place rather than be transported to a more secluded location, which can be a wooden area a block away, five feet around the wall of a building, a few feet from a walking path into the brush—anywhere that's out of sight. If an assailant want's to take you away, he's not a thief. He's after something else—access to your body, your life, or both. It gets violent and your odds become stacked against you.

Some individuals are afraid to make the attacker angry by not following his requests. They believe that if they do as they're told, they won't get hurt. However, if the criminal will hurt you in a public setting, what do you think he's going to do to you in private? You're likely better off taking the risk in a public location.

You never know what or who else is waiting for you at the second location but it's definitely not going to be in your favor. If an aggressor can't do what he want's to do at the first spot of contact, it's an indication that he want's to get you to a more isolated place; where the chances of being seen or heard are dramatically reduced. Never go to the second location. Do everything in your power to get out of the situation.

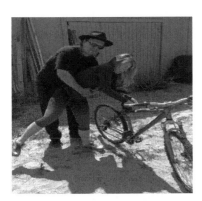

If an assailant want's to take you away to a secluded location he's after something else—access to your body, your life, or both.

Responding Intelligently and Responsibly

Making a decision to defend yourself involves some responsibility. That means you have to weigh-out the potential destructive ability of your assailant very quickly. Of course, if he brandishes a knife, gun, or similar deadly weapon, that immediately escalates the situation. He's showing you his clear intent to injure you with a deadly weapon. In that case, you'll likely be seen as justified (by the laws in your state) if you use all means at your disposal to fight for your life.

However, if a three year old child tried to slap you, you're naturally not going to claw their eyes out or break their knee. Likewise, if your best friend got drunk and went to push your shoulder, you similarly wouldn't go to immobilize them either. But if a 300 pound man suddenly blocks the only doorway you have to get out of your secluded warehouse office and suddenly morphs into a knife-wielding attacker, then all bets are off.

Obviously, all verbal confrontations should be avoided and deescalation should be the first option explored. Leaving the area, even if it means looking silly, should be pursued before things escalate into something more dangerous. It's always better to swallow your pride to keep yourself and your family safe. You can always release your annoyance within the safety of your own home, preferably by reevaluating the situation and blowing off steam by exercising or practicing the drills found in this book.

Don't Underestimate Your Abilities

If you think that you're not strong enough, tall enough, in-shape enough, or young enough to inflict serious damage and even death on your assailant, consider that some individuals have lifted cars that weighted a ton to release trapped loved ones underneath. The truth is that you don't know exactly what you're capable of until you have a burning desire. Your motivation is the key.

For example, if your leg flexibility level allowed you to bend forward to only touch your knees and someone offered you ten dollars to gain the flexibility to touch your toes in one month, you may not be motivated to even try. But if you were offered a million dollars to achieve the same task in the same amount of time you'd probably make sure that you accomplished it. The difference would be your motivation, your desire.

Your body may surprise you when your mind focuses its power of intent. That power of intent is unleashed by your motivation. With the right desire people have been known to accomplish seeming miracles. The point is to not underestimate your talents or your ability in self defense situations. Your mental power coupled by the skills you can achieve with practice and preparation will only help you in times of need.

Exploring Martial Arts and Other Combat Systems

A number of martial art systems have been around for thousands of years and are rich in history and tradition. Most advocate the valiant principles of discipline, respect, honor, persistence, and humbleness. There's great value in pursuing martial arts if you enjoy and gain physical and mental benefits from practicing them. With so many different styles available today, you can literally select those that make you happiest. Your martial arts class can challenge your cardiovascular system, increase your speed, and improve your accuracy and strength.

The challenge with martial arts is that people can sometimes get carried away and think that they're a super hero. Unfortunately, real life confrontations are vastly different from a controlled martial arts dojo environment. A real attacker won't stop short of punching you in the face or breaking your leg, unlike your considerate class partner. Likewise, you generally won't practice in your work attire in class, and instead will wear comfortable clothing and shoes.

Additionally, it's a good idea to explore different martial arts styles to test your strengths and weaknesses and to learn something new that helps you think outside the box.

In the same way that you memorize facts and figures (through years of repetition), when you practice movements through physical repetition your body stores the information into its "muscle memory." You then have a tendency to naturally react in the manner that you've been practicing. That's why it's wise to be selective about the motions you want to "ingrain" into your muscle memory.

Ideally, you want to program movements that will be practical to your self defense. Practicing, for example, doing a backward cartwheel to get away from an attacker (while looking good in the movies) may not be practical, even if it's fun for you.

Those practicing the same martial arts for many years tend to respond to the same angles of motion that their training partners throw. One art, for example, may focus on straight punches that go directly to the target (you) and you may get used to blocking those angles of attack for ages. That's why it's not uncommon for advanced practitioners to be sucker-punched by class beginners who use unconventional angles of attack the advanced person is not used to countering.

The more realistic your training, the better it is for you. So train with all sorts of people of different ages, shapes, and sizes. Be familiar with all angles of attack, especially those most unexpected. If you're used to perfect form and exact angles of attack and defense in your class, realize that you won't find that in a street situation. That's like thinking that you'll find perfectly made-up "model" looking people finishing a marathon instead of exhausted, dehydrated, and worn-out looking people. It's not reality.

Enjoy your martial arts classes and use them for your betterment. But don't expect that you'll have your sword, stick, or pole with you on the street, on the bus, or on a plane.

Remember, if you're forced into a battle with an assailant, understand that it's not a picnic—it's serious business. When you fight for your survival, the last thing on your mind will be thoughts of acting like a kung-fu star or yelling: "I got you sucker!" When you escape from an attacker you won't want to see that person for the rest of your life.

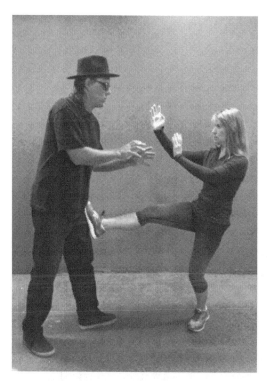

It's unlikely that you'll perform the perfect martial arts routine in a real self defense situation unless you're a highly trained expert.

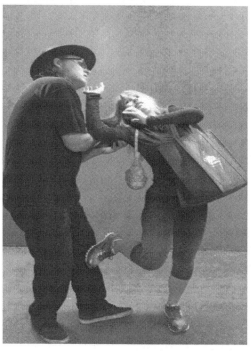

In reality you may be caught off guard while carrying items and being distracted, and may have to defend yourself from an awkward position while the assailant pulls out all the stops of fair-play including pulling your hair or having his buddies help him outnumber you.

Never Give Up

A Minneapolis woman was recently attacked at 4 p.m. in a
parking garage by an assailant who "camouflaged" himself
in a business suit. Because she was used to seeing men
dressed in business wear, she didn't think there was
anything unusual or out-of-place about him. She was
parked a few steps away from the elevator and was on her
way from work to school. As she was getting into her car,
the well-dressed man came up behind her and put a knife to
her throat. At first, she thought it was some kind of joke,
until she grabbed the blade and sliced her hand. She then
heard him say: "We're going for a ride." In that split-
second, she made a decision to fight for her life.

     She'd taken a self defense course at a local High
School and remembered a few strikes that she had learned.
She began stomping at the attackers feet, clawing at this
face, biting at his hand, and jabbing for his groin—while
kicking and screaming. During the three minutes that she
fought for her life, she tried unsuccessfully to remove the
bottle of repellant that she had in her purse. Though she
suffered a deep cut to her abdomen which reached her back
muscles, she didn't give up and escaped with her life. As
the assailant was fleeing, she heard him say: "You're lucky
you're a fighter." She now campaigns to bring awareness
about women's safety.[1] Because she saw a man who was
dressed in a business suit, she wasn't' alerted to danger.
Because she fought for her life and didn't give up, she got
away. Her attacker was later arrested—a lifelong predator
who went to great lengths to attack people by disguising
himself.

     Even in the most dire of circumstances, you should
never give up. If you're caught in the position where a

predator transports you to a secluded location, it's still not too late. If you are remotely capable of moving you can gouge his eyes, bite, and use everything in your power to escape. Focus on your survival and never give up.

Mental Self Defense

In some respects, much of the information contained in this book can be viewed as a part of mental self defense. Don't we engage in mental self defense when we choose to eat well to protect both our body and mind? Aren't we invoking mental self defense when we use discipline and determination to practice physical drills that increase our safety? What about the variety of techniques and tools found in this book that open up a conversation with ourselves and inspire new thoughts and ideas that we would not otherwise have considered; don't those also fall into the mental self defense category? Indeed, both our awareness and the decisions that we choose to make begin in our mind; and are vital lines of defense and protection against threats.

One of the reasons that an attacker is usually one step ahead of his intended target is because he has the element of surprise in his favor. His chosen target often does not even know that she (or he) is a target. Most never consider how to react and end up frozen or panicked. On the contrary, an assailant has put some thought into figuring out a strategy to accomplish his diabolical goals; while the target typically has put no thought at all into an escape or survival plan. This gives the assailant a mental edge.

However, we can take that edge away from an aggressor and give it to ourselves by mentally preparing ahead of time. We do this beforehand by figuring out the possible moves he can make and how to counter them in ways that benefit us most. Yes, it's similar to a game of chess, but with much higher stakes.

Think Like an Assailant (temporarily)

It's perfectly normal for those of us without any intention of ever harming others to have a difficult time visualizing ourselves as an assailant. It may be hard to put yourself in the aggressors shoes. You may think that it's a bad thing to do, that it makes you somehow evil too. It doesn't.

Temporarily making yourself the aggressor allows you to see the assailants goals from his perspective, which helps you detect where you're most vulnerable. You can then prepare yourself better for what may come next. In a profoundly practical way, you take the aggressors edge away from him and give it to yourself.

Some of the ways you can practice seeing things from the perspective of the aggressor is imagining where it would be easiest to attack others, particularly yourself, during the day. Are you most vulnerable when you leave the house, sleepy-eyed while holding a cup of coffee? Are you most tuned-out when you've finished work and can't see anything but that dinner that you plan on making? Only you know best when and where you're most vulnerable, so that in itself gives you more of an advantage. Since knowledge is power, once you become aware of your weaknesses, you can turn them into strengths.

Overcome Your Fear

Fear is a normal emotion that has the intended purpose of keeping us from danger. When put to good use, fear can be quite helpful, but when used indiscriminately, fear can be immobilizing and counterproductive; especially when we're already in danger and need to act quickly.

Too much fear has a way of throwing our mind and body out of balance. It can become the wrench thrown into a smoothly functioning mind; a mind that needs to be at its most effective during challenging confrontations. Fear, a close cousin of adrenaline, can rattle our equilibrium, which is something we can't afford too much of in a self defense situation.

What makes unexpected attacks so gut-wrenchingly frightening is being caught off guard. Being startled and shocked often causes the mind to freeze, which can cause hesitation and waste precious seconds that can be put to better use—like delivering aggressive opposition that will throw your assailant off guard and allow you to escape to safety. Turning the tables quickly on an assailant who least expects it puts him at a disadvantage and may cause him to hesitate or panic.

One of the biggest ways to overcome fear is to acknowledge that it exists and deal with it. Running away from fear won't help. An attacker will often try to intimidate us into fear, knowing that fear causes us to make hasty, and less than perfect decisions. That's why cultivating a different frame of mind often helps to stop fear in its tracks and gives us an edge. What frame of mind is that? The idea that the assailant should be afraid of you instead of you being afraid of him. Changing your attitude from: "I'm going to hurt him," to "I'm going to stop him" is often helpful for visualization purposes. When you focus on stopping the aggressor it takes your mind away from your fear, and gives you something constructive to center your attention on.

Remember, an assailant can keep attacking if he's merely hurt, but when his knee is shattered by a kick and he can't walk, or he can't see you because you clawed his eyes, then you have a better chance of escaping. Predators rarely quit if they're determined to inflict harm or worse so you need to render them *nonfunctional*, which means he can't move effectively—or even better—at all.

An assailant has a certain amount of confidence that he will be successful in his attack. He's probably scoped you out and sized up the kind of defense or compliance he's likely to get from you. When he does attack, he's expecting to have success. Imagine his shock and disappointment when he encounters an individual who's ready to tear his head off. Now he's scared for his own safety. You essentially turn the tables on him with your attitude, strength, and determination.

It's helpful to cultivate the mentality of turning on a "switch" within yourself that turns you into a person who's even more "dangerous" than your assailant. If it helps you to visualize that you have an "on" and "off" switch that gets triggered if you get attacked then you can use that for visualization purposes too.

Visualize to Gain the Edge

Top professional athletes are often trained to visualize successful outcomes of their movements. Many acclaimed golfing-greats have written extensively about their ability to imagine their hole-in-one hundreds of times before ever stepping onto the course. Thankfully, most of us visualize as part of our daily life without even consciously thinking about it.

Many individuals avoid contemplating potentially dangerous encounters because it brings up fear and anxiety. Sure, it may not be the most pleasant way to spend your time, but it could certainly be one of the most productive and effective in the context of improving your and your family's safety.

When you practice the kind of response you want to deliver in a confrontation beforehand in your minds-eye, you gain confidence and a greater ability to stay focused during some of the most stressful situations you may encounter in life. Visualization helps you imagine the actions you would take ahead of time in a variety of situations, saving valuable time in the future because you've already considered your options and responses with a clear mind, helping you accomplish that successful outcome in the future.

Mental imagery affects your fine motor coordination, attention, planning, perception, memory, motivation, and encourages your brain to get trained for the actual performance that you imagined. If you apply the same concepts to your self defense practice, your chances of success can increase as well.

One of the best times to visualize reacting to self defense situations is during the functional fitness drills that will be introduced in the following chapters. As you hit the target, which may be a medicine ball or a focus mitt, imagine that you're really striking an attacker. The more you visualize these types of scenarios vividly and with confidence, the more you increase your chances of reacting in exactly this way if your skills are ever called into action. Your body will automatically take over because of practice.

Visualizing reactions to different scenarios can be practiced at any time. Imagine what actions you would take if a predator started climbing through your window right now. Would you run? Where? As you contemplate your actions, keep focused on your breath. Do you find that you're holding your breath because of tension? See if you can relax and breathe deeply. Now try the scenario again. Do you feel just a bit calmer after you visualized it once? If you visualized it twenty times, would you feel even calmer and less panicked? This is the power of visualization–it helps you to react in ways that you desire in the future so you gain greater composure, confidence, and performance, and are less immobilized by fear.

Countering Scary Scenarios in Your Mind

A functional mental self defense exercise that can be practiced just about anywhere is imagining scary situations in your mind and responding to them effectively. Certain scenarios may be obviously recognized as dangerous, while others require more finesse and conscious discernment.

See yourself at various locations that you expect to find yourself during the day. Visualize yourself in your driveway as you're getting into your car. See yourself in the elevator going up to your office. Imagine yourself in your workplace cafeteria reading a book. Visualize you're in the parking lot walking to your car. See yourself enter your home at the end of the day. Visualize responding with quick and effective action for every scenario that you imagine.

It's possible that when you read each scenario, your mind may draw a blank and you may need some additional ideas to draw from. If that's the case, consider the method of logic and the stream of questions that you may ask yourself about each situation.

As you're getting out from behind the wheel of your car in a parking lot, you notice a man watching you from behind a nearby bench. He's crouching down; using the bench to conceal himself. What would you do?

Questions to consider:

- How do I feel? Does my intuition tell me to get back in the car, lock the doors, and drive away quickly?

- Where am I? Am I at a deserted park? Am I in a crowded area packed with people? Am I across the street from my house complex?

- Am I alone right now or do I have the company of several people who are also getting out of the car with me?

- If I'm only with my child (who I need to get out of their car seat), what's the distance between us and the man? Do I have enough time to escape with my child if I see the man aggressively approach us?

- Do I suddenly see a young child running towards the man yelling, "I found you daddy?" That could help explain this odd scenario.

- Do I see other men hanging around and getting closer to my car?

- Your own inquiry to consider adding here.

As you're carrying your groceries up the stairs to your apartment you hear the stairway door one floor below you open and shut. You hear someone start to run aggressively up the stairs behind you. What would you do?

Questions to consider:

- What time is it? Is it 5 p.m. when people are coming home from work and kids are running ahead of their parents to get home quickly, or is it 2 a.m. in the morning where it's very out of the norm for anyone to be aggressively running up the stairs?

- Will glancing down quickly to see if it's a neighbor help me or would my time be better spent quickly exiting on the nearest floor, where people may be home who can hear me if there's a confrontation?

You notice the guy at the gym who's been staring at you during your workout is now following you to your parked car. What would you do?

Questions to consider:

- Did this guy give me a bad vibe at the gym?

- Did this guy "case" out my stature and physical abilities more than just look at me out of mere curiosity?

- What is he wearing? Is it shorts and a T-shirt with no noticeable pockets or bulges or is it clothing that can conceal weapons?

- Is this parking lot outside in an open and crowded area or is it in a closed and secluded basement?

- Do I want this guy to see the car I drive and what's inside (if he chooses to scope it out later to gain more information about me)?

- Is he walking toward me and gaining speed to close the gap quickly or is he hovering back simply to see what I'm driving?

- Do I feel that I have enough distance to safely get in my car and drive away or will he be able to push me into my car when I open the door?

Your doorbell rings late at night and you're not expecting anyone. What would you do?

Your friend couldn't make it to meet you at the bar at the last moment, but you've had a few drinks while waiting and now you're alone and slightly tipsy. What would you do?

You're alone in the elevator when the door opens and a man gets in. You're a few floors away from your destination and he begins to edge his way closer to you. What would you do?

A well-dressed man approaches your car as you're sitting at a stop light during rush-hour traffic and you're not sure of his intent. What would you do?

You hear odd noises outside your bathroom door when you're in the shower and you live alone. What would you do?

You're by yourself in a public women's bathroom brushing your hair in front of the mirror and a man walks in. What would you do?

Your car breaks down in a rural section of town, where there's no phone reception, and no one is around. What would you do?

A man is walking towards you with "Lost Dog" fliers as you're taking an early morning walk in your neighborhood; you've never seen him before. What would you do?

Continue to challenge yourself with your own scenarios to build your confidence and self empowerment.

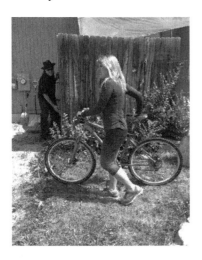

Visualization helps you imagine the actions you would take ahead of time in a variety of situations, saving valuable time in the future because you've already considered your options and responses with a clear mind, helping you accomplish that successful outcome in the future.

Acting for Your Life

Most people who lack the predator mindset are naturally honest and forthcoming. However, when you're dealing with an attacker who's intent on doing you harm, you must throw out all your courtesy, manners, and sense of honesty away to increase your chances of survival. That means you may have to be prepared to lie and cheat to save your life.

It's perfectly fine to use every underhanded element you can think of to encourage the predator to underestimate you. The more he underestimates you the greater your advantage. Predators have no "rules" of conduct or engagement–they'll do anything to attain their goal. So all bets should be off if you're being assaulted. Your mental framework must change in an instant from a kind, gentle person, to a warrior who will do anything to survive.

Psychology must come in when survival is at stake. While martial arts and other self defense modalities teach you the fighting arts, the one thing they don't actively teach you is *acting*.

That's why it's beneficial to learn how to "act" to a predator since some women have escaped by talking their way out of a situation. There have been instances where a man had his clothes off ready to assault a woman and she "pretended" to agree with the situation. The acting bought her additional time to grab a weapon or escape to safety. The key to practicing your acting is using your visualization skills (discussed earlier).

Visualize your attitude, your demeanor, how you would act in various situations if you're confronted. How would your face look? If you had to pretend to go along with an aggressors demands, could you make it look believable for an instant to throw him off guard?

Don't underestimate your ability to act and use it to your full advantage in a dangerous situation.

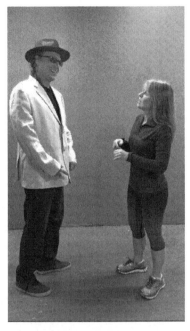

An assailant has no reservations about using acting to gain the upper hand. He may initially approach you as a "good guy" who want's to be friendly, which may lower your guard and make you feel comfortable around him.

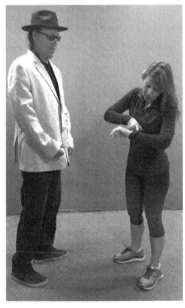

It's not uncommon for an assailant to use distraction tactics like asking you for the time or directions to well known local landmarks. This makes him appear vulnerable and in need of your assistance.

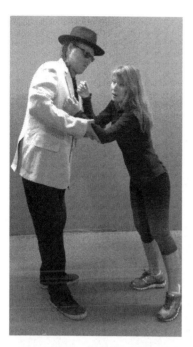

When an assailant sees his opportunity he may make his move, catching you off guard.

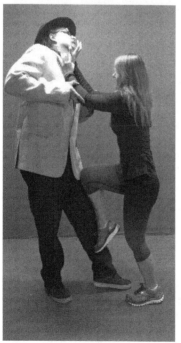

How you react will help determine your escape to safety.

Chapter 9

Tools, Targets, and Functional Fitness

Survival situations are not fair fights. Chances are great that if you're not actively causing injury to an attacker, then he is probably injuring you or dragging you to a secondary location. That's why it's important to practice striking targets that count ahead of time. The more you train, the higher your chances of hitting your mark; and an effective strike that incapacitates an attacker may mean the difference between a safe escape or not.

From a self defense perspective, you want to start thinking about your tools and targets. Tools are essentially weapons that can inflict bodily harm or physical damage to an attacker. We often think of guns, knives, or similar objects as weapons, but what about the fork you eat with? Can it be used as a weapon to spear the eyes or throat of an attacker? How about a scorching cup of coffee? That can become a weapon too, and so can a writing pen if it strikes an attackers eyes and vital targets.

When you start to cultivate a frame of mind that looks for things in your immediate environment as useful weapons, it helps you focus your mindset on successful survival. Weapons may help save your hands and fingers from damage during contact with hard body surfaces such as bones, since they're generally stronger and can take some punishment. They give you the extra edge that can help you escape from a threatening scenario quickly.

Noticing potential weapons that you commonly have on hand every day can tip the odds in your favor and helps cultivate a survival mindset.

Along with makeshift weapons, your body is a powerful and strong weapon. Of course, certain body parts are more conducive to striking and hitting than others. For example, it would be more advantageous for you to strike with your knee or foot, than your nose or neck for obvious anatomical reasons. While just about any part of your body can be used as a weapon, there are certain ones that are more effective in a self defense situation, especially if you know how to use them through practice and visualization.

What are the targets on an attackers body that you want to go after? The eyes, throat, groin, knee, and the top of the foot. The principle of "economy of motion," popularized by the legendary martial artist and philosopher Bruce Lee, encourages inflicting the most amount of damage in the shortest amount of time by going after targets that are closest to you. If an attackers face is the closest target, you'll strike that. If his foot is closer, you'll go for that. The goal is to keep things simple and straightforward because simple motions are remembered best in stressful situations which means they'll be most effective. The concepts presented in the next sections will help inspire more ideas and expand your self defense thought-process.

Overcoming the Fear of Hurting Someone

Before we discuss the tools that can inflict damage to an attacker and the best targets to aim for, it will be helpful to first ask yourself a few important questions, namely: Are you mentally prepared to harm someone who intends to assault or kill you (and your children)? What's your reaction when you visualize clawing an attackers eyes? Are you appalled at the thought? Do you wonder if you can do it?

Now imagine that an aggressor is dragging your small child away or that your elderly and frail grandmother is being assaulted. Do these scenarios help you to break through your fear and spur you into action? Does your hesitation suddenly disappear? Remember, you're not just hurting someone out of the blue because you feel like it. You're protecting your life and the lives of your family members against an aggressive criminal who's fully prepared to take your life and the lives of your loved ones.

An aggressor makes a decision to attack–you don't make that choice for him. He has to deal with the repercussions of his actions, which could mean his own demise. Criminals understand that they may get injured or killed during an assault or robbery situation and they're willing to take that risk. Holding back from unleashing your full self defense actions doesn't help you and only assists the attacker. That's why it's critical to overcome the fear of hurting your assailant.

One way is to do that is by using the visualization tools presented in this book. Visualization, along with your new mindset that says that you will not hesitate to act firmly when it comes to protecting yourself and your family will help you overcome your initial apprehension. Remember, assailants count on your fear, confusion, panic, and immobilization to get what they want. Don't let them.

The Tools

Any part of your body can become a powerful weapon, but there are certain areas that are more effective than others in certain situations because of their harder structure, flexibility, and range of motion. Take a look at the following partial list of body weapons you have at your disposal and remember that *anything* can be used as a weapon.

Your Conscious Decision to Ignore Pain—You must mentally prepare yourself for the fact that you're likely to get hurt in some way. It can be a tiny scratch or it can be much worse. Whatever injury you sustain during an attack, you must be mentally prepared to keep going. Cultivating this frame of mind is critically important. The adrenaline that your body will release during an attack situation will help numb some of the pain from any injuries that you may experience, but it's always helpful to decide beforehand that your pain will not distract you from your goal of getting away to safety.

Mental Awareness—Foremost, your mind is your best weapon. Good judgment, keen awareness, and a honed intuition can help you size up a situation in mili-seconds; helping you choose the best course of action. The more successful outcomes you visualize in advance to a wide range of scenarios (using the visualization techniques found in this book), the faster your mind will tend to come up with solutions in stressful situations.

Your Powerful Voice—Some martial arts employ a type of short, energetic "yell" before, during, or after executing a technique. The purpose of this yell is to startle and intimidate an opponent, expressing confidence and victory. By using mental imagery techniques, practitioners visualize the yell starting in their diaphragm (not the throat) and extending from there. Some highly skilled martial art masters can stun and even immobilize an opponent without even touching him simply by executing a powerful yell. For our purposes here, keep your powerful voice forefront in your mind, as it can deliver an intense yell that may not only momentarily disorganize an attacker, but also signal an alarm to others to come to your assistance. Be prepared to scream like never before. If you have access to a location that allows you to practice your yell without panicking others to call law enforcement, then certainly practice often. Other opportunities to yell are during roller-coaster rides and concerts. Gauge how quickly your voice volume decreases and how long it takes for your voice to give-out. See how fast your voice recovers again. Keeping these factors in mind ahead of time will give you a rough estimate of your voice capacity and propel you to practice. It's also a good idea to research ways of training your yell in ways that don't harm your vocal cords. Much of this information is readily available online or through books.

Teeth—Amazingly, our incisors can generate pounds of pressure, along with our molars, all from what we do every day—chew food! Biting is a very effective self defense technique, requiring only your teeth and the attackers exposed flesh. While it's generally not the first line of attack, biting down on a predators arm, hand, or any other protruding target should not be ignored if it presents itself in close vicinity of your mouth or if you're immobilized in a position from which you can't move. Bite down viciously and twist to cause maximum damage.

Elbows—An elbow to the nose, temple, throat, or other vulnerable body target can be devastating to an attacker. Since your elbow is mostly solid, it can make a tremendous impact on a soft target without sustaining too much damage. One way we all unconsciously perform elbow-style movements is when we put on our seat belt in the car or when we scratch our back. Practice elbow motions in the air or against a focus-pad and incorporate elbow strikes at close range when practicing the functional fitness drills in the following chapter.

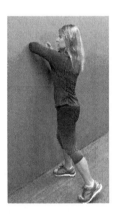

You can practice elbow placement motions against a wall to develop accuracy and familiarize yourself with the movements (without hitting the wall so you don't damage your elbow or the wall).

Fingers—Your fingers can be powerful scratching and clawing weapons. It's also a good idea to reevaluate having long nails as they can painfully break if a strike is made with your hand. The longer the nail, the more leverage it provides to pop right off your finger if it strikes an attackers body very hard. Additionally, long nails prevent proper fist closure since they dig into your palms. Fingers are often the last body part we work on strengthening, so it's practical to challenge them whenever the opportunity comes up. Some fun ways to develop finger strength includes kneading dough, opening and closing your fingers in the sand, and providing resistance to each finger as it opens and closes with the help of your opposite hand.

Knees—Striking an attacker in the groin with the knee can be very effective. Kneeing can inflict a tremendous amount of damage if done to a good target. Choice targets for kneeing include the face, groin, or the side of the thigh. If you executed an effective strike to an attackers eyes and he instinctively jerks forward instead of backwards, his face may come close to your knee. This is a good opportunity to knee his face quickly as you make your getaway. Keep in mind that it's almost impossible to knee effectively (or at all) while wearing constricting clothing that does not allow for sufficient leg movement.

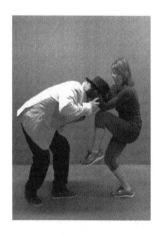

A knee to the face.

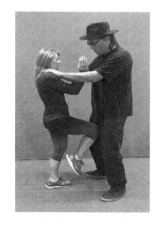

A knee to the groin.

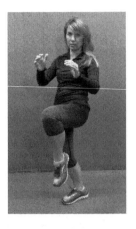

Practice knee drills at home to gain balance and accuracy.

Feet—Your feet are one of your best weapons. Low kicks are difficult for an attacker to see, especially if he's tall and not expecting them. Low kicks to the knee are also hard to block, and stomping on top of an aggressors foot with your full weight can injure him enough for you to flee to safety. While you may have the flexibility of a professional ballet dancer, it's generally best to avoid high-kicks in self defense situations. It's simply too easy for an attacker to grab your leg and pull you off balance; you can also slip easier. Kicking to a higher target means your foot must travel a greater distance to reach its intended target, which often takes more time; and you can also pull a leg muscle or tendon easier, causing you immediate pain and limiting your further movement. Is it worth kicking high considering the risks? Probably not. Think low kicks in self defense scenarios. Sure, high kicks can be fun at the gym or in the controlled and disciplined environment of a martial arts dojo; and they certainly look great in the movies. However, their practical use is often limited to high-level experts and, unless you are one, it's often best to keep your kicks low. Also, be conscious about your shoe choices as they can directly inhibit not only your means of escape, but also your balance should you choose to kick.

It's generally best to avoid high-kicks in self defense situations. It's simply too easy for an attacker to grab your leg and pull you off balance.

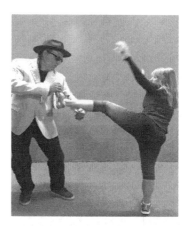

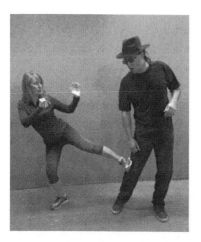

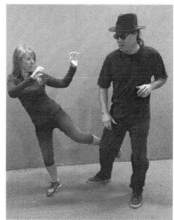

Low kicks are difficult for an attacker to see, especially if he's tall and not expecting them; they're also hard to block. A solid kick may injure him enough for you to flee to safety.

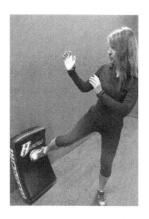

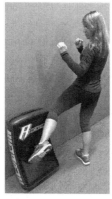

Practice low kicks at home against a kicking shield to develop balance, speed, and muscle memory, or have your partner hold a kicking shield to develop your power.

Forehead–Using your forehead to head-butt an attacker should not be your first choice of weapon–but it could be an option when few remain. Head-butting can be effective if executed quickly to a vulnerable target such as an aggressors nose if your arms are tied-up and you don't have many choices. Remember to use the hard part of your head, not your face. Head-butting should be trained in advance to gain some accuracy. If you're held from behind and your hands are tied-up, you can head-butt with the back of your head to an attackers nose if he's close to your height. Head-butting, of course, will not work well on a taller assailant as you'll hit his chest, which tends to be resilient.

The Targets

Unfortunately, many individuals have not been taught effective self defense skills, so when they're confronted by an assailant, they end up flailing their arms at the attackers chest or abdomen, which generally has little to no effect on him, especially if he has a large chest or abdomen.

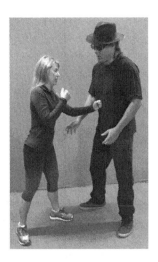

Punching an assailants chest or abdomen will likely have little effect on him and you may risk breaking your wrist or knuckles. Instead, focus your energy on vulnerable targets that damage the assailant.

While you may posses a mean and powerful punch, is it really smart to risk breaking your knuckles in a real confrontation? Survival is not a boxing match—the goal is to hit as many vulnerable targets on the attacker as possible in the shortest amount of time and escape quickly. This is why you want to go for the targets that count—those that will inflict the most damage to him—and the least amount of damage to you.

In an ideal scenario, you would want to stop your attacker so he is no longer a threat. Again, changing your frame of mind from: "I'm going to hurt him," to "I'm going to stop him" is often helpful for visualization purposes. Remember, an assailant can keep attacking if he's merely hurt, but when his knee is shattered by a kick he and he can't walk, or he can't see you because you clawed his eyes, then you may have a better chance of escaping.

The best way to improve your skills and accuracy level is through practice. Regardless of your fitness level, if you don't practice accuracy by hitting targets in a training setting, your chances of delivering an effective strike will decrease—especially when your life depends on it.

Also, you can't expect that your first strike will be effective. You must assume that it may not connect for a number of reasons: he may move out of range unexpectedly; you may lose your balance and miss; and he may absorb your strike without enough harm to cause him to stop the attack. So you must continually follow up with additional strikes until you can escape to safety. That's why keeping a focus on the attackers vital targets are so important.

While some view UFC matches as a no-holds-barred fight, they do have some rules, namely; the following (and more) moves are not allowed:

- Eye gouging
- Butting with the head
- Biting
- Hair pulling
- Groin attacks
- Throat strikes
- Clawing, pinching or twisting flesh
- Kicking the head
- Kneeing the head

Can you guess some of the reasons these moves are not allowed during full-contact fights which match some of the toughest, most hard-core professional fighters in the world? If you said it's because these maneuvers can cause severe, permanent damage or even death—effectively ending a fight quickly—you are correct.

While these moves are not allowed in the rink, they are *exactly* the movements you're looking for to defend your life. The following partial list of targets are important to keep in mind to better understand why striking them is so dangerous.

Eyes—If you take a glass cup and flick it with your finger, it won't feel very powerful—but would you want someone to do that to your eye? Merely getting a speck of dirt in our eye is painful and makes it difficult to see. Our eyes are so sensitive that even a stray eyelash or a piece of dust can cause severe watering and irritation. Now imagine getting hit in the eye with some force.

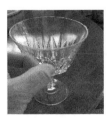

If you take a glass cup and flick it with your finger, it won't feel very powerful—but would you want someone to do that to your eye?

Eye strikes can leave an attacker temporarily blinded, allowing you to punch, kick, or run to safety. Effectively striking an aggressors eyes does not require years of training and it's an effective technique that can buy you time during a surprise attack. If an assailants eyes are damaged or injured, how well can he see? Even if you miss the eyes, he may blink (an automatic reaction) and this may give you an opportunity to follow up with a kick or another move. Even if your finger merely grazes one of his eyes, it will immediately water and his vision will severely blur. That's why the eyes are the number one target. Try to keep your jabbing fingers close to one another and slightly bent to avoid finger injury of the joints in case of accidental connection with the bony part of an assailants face. Make it a point to practice executing eye jabs at home on various targets or have a partner hold a tennis ball at your eye level and practice striking it with your fingers. A great deal of strength is not needed to accomplish an effective eye strike, but practice helps develop speed, accuracy, and a sense of timing, which are attributes you want, especially in a stressful situation. Avoid telegraphing an eye jab to an attacker to keep the element of surprise to your advantage.

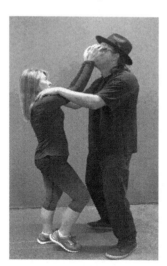

Effectively striking an aggressors eyes does not require years of training and it's an effective technique that can buy you time during a surprise attack.

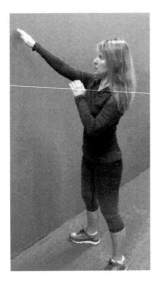

Make it a point to practice executing eye jabs at home on various targets.

Throat—The throat is an exposed body part that, once damaged, can restrict air passageways. If an assailant can't breathe adequately, how well will he be focused on running after you? The chances of him stopping an attack increase if he has his own survival to worry about. Since the throat is located lower than a persons eyes, it makes for a closer target for persons of a shorter stature who can't reach the eyes of a much taller attacker. You can practice striking the throat by having a partner hold a focus-pad or similar object, and visualize hitting the throat as you strike with the palm of your hand or the side of your hand in a chopping-style motion.

Knee—How well can an assailant run after you if his knee is broken or injured? Damaging a knee is similar to breaking one foot off a chair; it becomes unstable and can easily collapse. Kicking the knee with your foot is sometimes wise because it's often least expected and more difficult for an attacker to see since it's done below his line of vision. You can kick the side of the knee or the front; both inflict damage that is difficult to contend with. Practice a basic side kick at home, visualizing striking a predators knee. Try not to look down as this will telegraph your intent. Have a partner hold a kicking shield or pad low to the ground where a persons knee is located and practice kicking the target from both sideways and from the front.

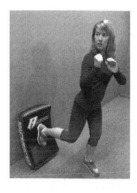

Practice striking the knee area of an imaginary assailant from all angles, including from behind you.

Foot—Using our body weight to stomp on an assailants foot can be very effective, especially if he's wearing flimsy shoes. Incapacitating the foot is always a painful distraction as walking becomes more difficult, if not impossible. The nerves on top of the foot are fragile and vulnerable; no amount of weight lifting will cushion or protect this area with extra muscle and bulk. Most shoes are not as reinforced or padded at the top as they are on the bottom since they have to step on concrete and other terrains. This makes the top of the foot vulnerable to damage in many cases. Striking your heel hard on top of an attackers foot means you have gravity (not to mention your full weight) working for you since you're motion is downward. Use those elements to your advantage.

Groin—The groin is a vulnerable target, and men have a tendency to protect it because they're aware that women generally have some idea that it's a target. Going for the groin is almost expected by some men, which means you may not have the same element of surprise as with other targets. Of course, if there is an opportunity to inflict damage to the groin–take it. Use your knee, foot, or hand. Grab and twist the groin with your hand; punch it, and use any weapons at your disposal to inflict damage. If the attacker moves his head forward when you connect with his groin, knee his face or rake his eyes.

The Element of Surprise

Have you ever been the happy recipient of a surprise party that you knew nothing about? When people jumped out and yelled, "Surprise!" did you get a little shocked and stunned? That's the kind of reaction you want to inflict on an aggressor who thinks you're going to be an easy target. But instead of a pleasant surprise, you want him to get the shock of his life by having the tables turned on him. He suddenly and unexpectedly has to worry about his own skin.

What you want to deliver is a *blindingly fast shock followed by intense pain* so you can escape to safety. The kind of pain that's immobilizing. The kind of pain that makes harming you or your loved ones the last thing on his criminal mind. And even if your harm is still on his agenda, it's going to be very hard to accomplish now that he can't see clearly, or from the loss of use of one of his legs. You effectively render the weapon (the assailant) temporarily harmless (always assume he can be faking an injury to get you to drop your guard). That's the combination you're looking for. His shock and intense, immobilizing pain. Your success. Your escape. Your safety.

When do you stop striking? When you feel you can safely get away. If the assailant can still come after you, assume that he will.

Ideally, you want to avoid showing all your "cards" to an attacker because the goal is to stun him with the element of surprise. Throwing an aggressor off-balance with a quick reaction and a flurry of vicious hits is using your mind and body to your best advantage. Of course, if there's enough time and you have the distance available to you—it's best to escape to a safer location. But if the attack is sudden and at close range, you need the element of surprise in your favor—not his. A lightning fast response to a violent attack is like throwing water on a fire: *you fizzle his momentum.* You can also think of it as "taking the wind out of his sails," the air out of his balloon, and so on. Discouragement is psychologically defeating and is the first step toward winning over your attacker.

The advantage that an aggressor commonly has on his side is the element of surprise—he's in control of when he's going to attack and how—and you don't have that information. So you must anticipate a wide range of scenarios to give yourself the advantage of a fast reaction. That's where visualization and practice come in; they instill a fast and trained automatic response in you that kicks into gear when it's called for. Most aggressors don't expect quick, fierce, and effective opposition. They expect to dominate and win what they want. If they didn't have that confidence, chances are that they'd look for an easier target. So when you become a vortex of violent fury, you effectively turn the tables on him—now he's on the defense. Also keep in mind that an attacker can have accomplices in the shadows ready to help him, so always remain alert for additional criminals who work in teams.

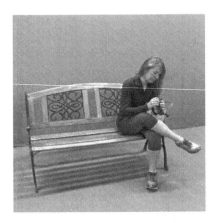

Always be aware and alert.

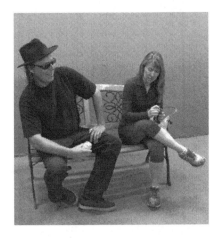

A seemingly safe scenario can escalate into a very dangerous one in mere seconds.

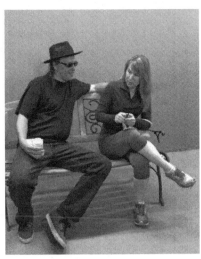

You can choose to get up and move away to a safer location if you feel that your personal space is being threatened.

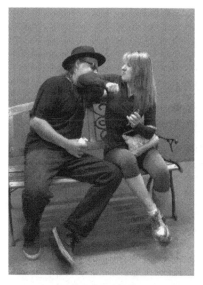

If an attack is made against you before you have a chance to escape, you can elbow an assailants vital target as you get away.

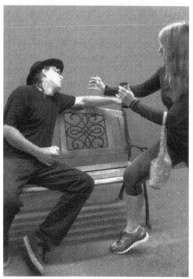

Remember to back-shuffle first before you run away in case the assailant goes to grab you from behind.

Anticipate a wide range of scenarios to give yourself the advantage of a fast reaction. If there's enough time and you have the distance available to you–it's best to escape to a safer location. But if the attack is sudden and at close range, you need the element of surprise in your favor–not his.

Responding to Violent Moves

The following scenarios are simply some ideas to get you thinking about possible reactions to common attacker moves. Keep in mind that these are merely concepts; each individual encounter will have countless variables that will require a unique response to that situation.

The Back-Shuffle—If a potential assailant makes a move towards you and you believe that you may be in danger but you're not sure, there are a number of options available. If you're simply looking for a bit of distance because you're not certain of his intent (he's drunk) and you're in a situation with lots of people around (still not a guarantee that they will come to your aid), you can do a back-shuffle. Simply stand with one leg forward and angle your body slightly. Then, as naturally as it feels to your body, shuffle backwards like someone is moving toward you to step on your toes. Keep your posture upright and your eyes forward on the person (or imaginary target) in front of you, while staying aware to the obstacles and people around you. Practice back-shuffling at home, in your gym, and at bootcamp (some bootcamps practice footwork moves). It's a critically important move to practice since most of us walk forward and we rarely move backward or laterally. A back-shuffle allows you some space and a little time to evaluate a situation before you make a decision. Sometimes that's all it takes to gain some safe distance between an adversary and then sprint out of there.

The Bridge—The Bridge is an important move if you don't have the room to back shuffle away from an attacker because of a wall or another obstacle. The Bridge becomes a partial barrier that helps protect your face and puts you in a "ready" position. When you put up your arm up and slightly bend it at the elbow, you create a bridge. From that point, a decision needs to be made. Can you run? If not, it may be a good idea to strike the attackers eyes or throat. If his hand is in the way, push it aside and go for his vulnerable targets.

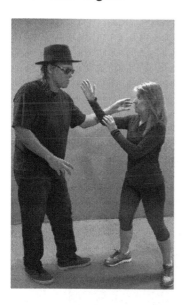

The Bridge. Do your best to keep your hands up when your personal space is threatened so your hands are in a better position to defend yourself. Keeping your hands up also makes them closer to your assailants vital targets so you'll reach them faster.

Choke from Behind—If you're caught off-guard and an assailant chokes you from behind, the main threats are your loss of consciousness due to the pressure exerted on the carotid artery, and the cutoff of air flow from your trachea. If possible: turn your head towards his elbow. If your chin can temporarily find the groove between his elbow you'll have slightly more air to buy you a bit of time. Grab his hand with one of your hands and bite him if you can, while at the same time work at clawing his face with your other hand while you stomp his feet. Chokes from behind are common when an attacker has a van or car parked close by ready to transport you away. It's sometimes easier to force a smaller person into a van by using a choke since your body must naturally follow where you're head is going and your attention is focused on trying to breathe more than anything. Do you very best to avoid being snuck up on behind your back. Always be alert for people who stand behind you and the potential of a choke from behind.

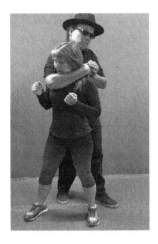

If possible: turn your head towards his elbow. If your chin can temporarily find the groove between his elbow you'll have slightly more air to buy you a bit of time.

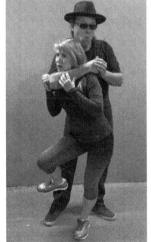

Grab his hand with one of your hands and bite it if you can, while at the same time work at clawing his face with your other hand while you stomp his feet.

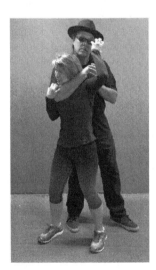

The Mount—If you find yourself on your back, either because you were pushed or lost your balance; or you woke up to an assailant who's now trying to choke or punch you, chances are good that he has or will try to "mount" you. That simply means he will try to sit on you with your body between his legs to try to pin you down for more control. But that may also put him at a certain disadvantage too. First, it may leave your arms free and within hitting range of his throat. If he leans forward his eyes may become available. This is the time to bring your hands up and claw like crazy. Thumb-gouge his eyes by inserting your thumbs into his eye sockets and pull outwards. If his glasses are in the way, strike under the eyes. If you're clawing really fast, those glasses will fly off. If you can't get to his eyes, use your fingers to strike his throat. (You can also chop the throat with either side of your hand, preferably the outside). You'd be surprised at just how strong your gluteus muscles are. You can throw a man off balance by mimicking a common exercise: Simply lay down flat on your back and "buck" your hips as if you're thrusting up. Practice this motion with your training partner or a trusted friend. See how fast they fly forward and become unbalanced when you "buck" your hips up. This is an exercise you can practice every day. As you progress, place a medicine ball or weights on your hips and practice the motion, gradually increasing the weight. Practicing will help you get used to bucking instinctively and it will come more naturally to you in a situation if needed.

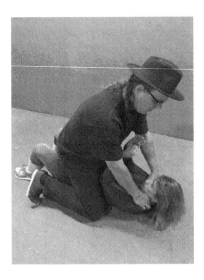

You can throw an assailant off balance by mimicking a common exercise: Simply lay down on your back and "buck" your hips as if you're thrusting up. Practice this motion with your training partner or a trusted friend. See how fast they fly forward and become unbalanced when you "buck" your hips up.

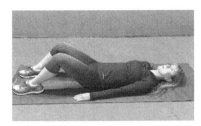

This is an exercise you can practice every day. Simply lay down on your back and "buck" your hips as if you're thrusting up.

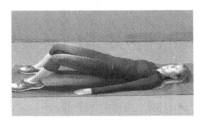

Practicing will help you get used to bucking instinctively and it will come more naturally to you in a situation if needed.

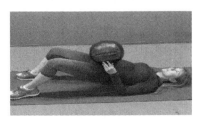

As you progress, place a medicine ball or weights on your hips and practice the motion, gradually increasing the weight.

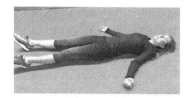

If possible, avoid falling backwards as shown to help prevent the back of your head from hitting the ground.

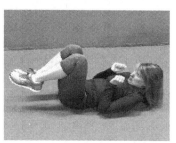

Instead, if you're pushed or lose your balance and fall backwards, try to keep your chin tucked close to your chest to protect the back of your head from hitting the ground, and keep your hands up to protect your face.

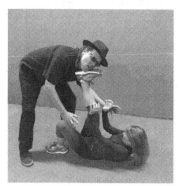
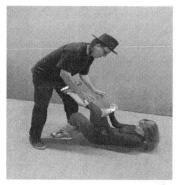

Keep your knees bent so your legs can be used to kick the assailants vital targets if he attempts to mount or strike you.

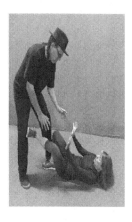

Keep your hands up, your chin close to your chest to avoid hitting your head against the ground, and use your powerful legs to deliver strikes to his knees or other valuable targets. Deliver strikes to the assailant as he gets within your range. If he tries to circle around you, turn your body to follow him and keep your (fighting weapons) legs between you. Be extra alert for additional attackers who may approach you from other directions.

Grabs—Some of the most common moves an assailant may attack with is various types of grabs. It's instinctual to try to resist grabs, naturally pulling our hand away like we would from a hot stove. But with a larger and stronger assailant, trying to wrestle your wrist or arm away may be futile and waste precious energy and time. If an aggressor grabs your wrist and attempts to drag you somewhere (into an auto, behind the bushes, into a house); instead of fighting against his power, go with him momentarily while inflicting damage to his available vital targets (eyes, throat, groin, knee) with your available hand or foot. (He may also adjust and use his hold to keep you away from him rather than pulling you towards him). Use any forward momentum that you may have to give you the additional power to cause damage to his vulnerable targets. If he's simply holding your wrist and you want to get lose, twist your wrist and hand toward his thumb, which is the weakest spot of his hold. If he follows your motion, hit his elbow forward with your other hand while breaking the grasp.

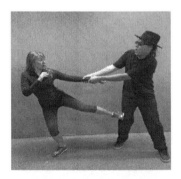

If an aggressor grabs your wrist and attempts to drag you somewhere; instead of fighting against his power, go with him momentarily while inflicting damage to his available vital targets (eyes, throat, groin, knee) with your available hand or foot.

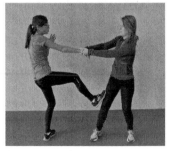

Practice grabbing your partner and having them strike the vital targets such as a knee.

214

Use His Momentum—If an attacker is trying to pull you, more than likely he will be physically stronger than you. Use his pulling momentum to strike your foot into his knee. Take his energy and use it against him. You can then claw his eyes with one of your hands if he keeps pulling. A familiar saying in some martial arts is: If he pulls, you push. If he pushes, you pull. That simply means that instead of trying to fight power with power (you may have much less than your aggressor), you simply use his power against himself. If he tries to punch you (a kind of a push) make sure your face moves away from where he expects his strike to land and use his forward momentum to drive your foot into his knee. It's similar to a car crash. If car number one is traveling at a certain speed and hits a stable, unmoving target it will have a fixed amount of damage. But if two cars are traveling toward each other at the same speed, the damage will be magnified because they're both moving. The idea is to use your attackers momentum to your advantage. Strike forward as he's moving forward. If he retreats see if you have the distance to safely escape.

Don't Turn Your Back Too Soon—When you strike an attackers eyes or throat and he's goes down on the ground, make sure you do a back shuffle before you turn around to run away. If you strike (and he's still close) and you turn to run too soon, you may set yourself up for a choke from the back or to have you hair pulled and be dragged down. Keep your eyes on the assailant after you strike him; then gauge your distance and then get out of there. Ideally, you want to continue to strike until the assailant is incapacitated but certain situations may dictate that you don't have that luxury; you may be too injured to continue; you may have an injured loved one who needs you to call for assistance quickly; and there are thousands of scenarios where you won't be able to guarantee that the assailant will stay down for any length of time. You can only do your best in each situation, so stay alert for the attackers recovery as you run away or call for assistance. That's why physical practice and visualization *ahead of time* are so effective in stressful situations; they increase your odds by giving you the physical and mental skills you wouldn't have otherwise had; instilling a frame of mind that's conducive to survival. Your survival mindset.

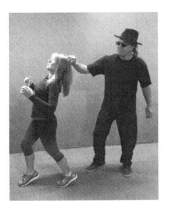

Don't turn your back too soon to the assailant. If you strike him (and he's still close) and you turn to run too soon, you may set yourself up for a choke from the back or to have your hair pulled to be dragged down.

Functional Fitness

Have you been influenced by the fitness industry to do hundreds of repetitions with tiny dumbbells? Were you ever tempted to buy the latest gimmicky fitness equipment with names similar to the Butt Toner, Thigh Slimmer, Chest Booster, Chin Trimmer, Waist Firmer, and other products because of the promises in those mesmerizing commercials? You're hardly alone.

We all want the magical gadgets that we think will give us instant results, but life simply doesn't work that way. Unfortunately, working out without sufficient weights fails to provide the challenge we really need to increase our strength. Neither does performing thousands of repetitions with apparatuses that hold little functional value. For example, the Butt Booster (a made up name of an imaginary product) will not help you get in and out of a chair or a toilet with ease throughout your lifetime, and it certainly won't assist you when functionality really counts −in real-life self defense scenarios. However, a squat will because it's a functional movement. If you want to stay healthy, fit, and be able to perform self defense motions under stress, then *you must practice functional movements*.

Many workout machines fail in their ability to provide practical and functional movements because they mimic the common postures that we perform all day long: sitting or laying down. In the real world, you'll probably face an attacker standing up (at least initially) so you must use your body in a more fluid way. That's why it's important to develop the ability to both push and pull (an aggressor), along with the learned skill of mobilizing yourself quickly−that initial explosive reaction that you want if you're confronted by an assailant.

When you imitate practical self defense movements in your work out; throwing a medicine ball becomes similar to doing a standup push-up; and throwing the medicine ball against the wall can mimic a punch or palm strike, just like in boxing because the gross movements are closely related. That means you can take your fitness workout and turn it into something functional for self defense. It's a win-win. You get an amazingly challenging training session while simultaneously honing your self defense skills.

The aim is to ingrain practical movements into your neurological system so the moves become reflexive, where you don't have to think about them consciously any more.

They'll automatically come out when you need them—but only if you practice or visualize the movements regularly.

Take a look at the following suggestions on how to add functional fitness into your day.

- It's a great idea to join a boot camp or do Cardio-Kick boxing where you're challenged to work on lateral motions, quick footwork, and punching and kicking. You can practice these motions in the air at home (sometimes called shadow-boxing). All these movements can come to your aid when you need them and you also get the added bonus of challenging your brain, which increases your cognitive fitness.

- Have a partner hold a boxing pad for you and go all out on it, clawing and gouging it as fast and hard as you can. Note how that feels. Visualize a real live attacker in front of you, not just a striking pad. This is a functional drill that may help you in a tough situation.

- Get used to being jarred slightly in a training setting so you're not shocked or thrown off guard if you experience such motions in a self defense situation. Get used to what it feels like to get grabbed in a safe training environment. Focus on reacting quickly and decisively, with as much speed and power as you can muster.

- If you get hit in the street and go down, you need the motion of being able to push back up quickly, so it's perfectly fine to do a bench press at home or at the gym, work with machine cables, or do a military press with weights that are really challenging.

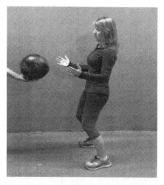

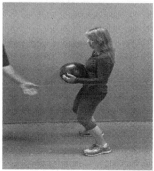

Throw a medicine ball back and forth with a partner and allow it to hit you in the abdominal region a bit as you catch it. Tighten your core as the ball moves towards you. This gets your body used to being "tagged" slightly and at your own pace, so that if you're punched in a self defense situation at least you'll have a bit of an idea of what it feels like to get hit because your body will have felt it in a controlled situation. This may help you later to stay focused rather that be shocked because you've been hit.

- Practice grabbing a workout partners hands and pulling and pushing each other. Sensitivity drills inherent to martial arts such as wing chun and tai chi, where the hands stay connected and you can feel the other persons motions, are also practical, fun, and deliver an intense workout.

Training for the "Adrenaline Dump"

Did you ever get so startled or scared that you "froze up?" Your body suddenly couldn't move, even though you wanted to. You may have felt weak, queazy, and sweaty during this time or immediately after. There are important reasons for this.

Our body has an inherent fight-or-flight mechanism built into it. In the past, if we were confronted by danger in the wild we could fight, run away, or sometimes freeze (hoping to look docile and not be perceived as a threat −handy if we accidentally stumbled on mama bear who was protecting her cubs).

When we perceive a dangerous situation, adrenaline is released in our body. That's often a good thing as adrenaline makes us less sensitive to pain; in case we're injured so we can keep going longer. Blood flow is also pulled away from our extremities in case of injury and more oxygen is provided to our heart and lungs so we can run with more stamina without getting tired quickly. But adrenaline messes with our fine motor coordination and our thinking processes; our ability to make clear and rash decisions is also compromised. Those are not the attributes we want in a self defense situation. So when you're confronted with an assailant intent on doing you harm or taking your life, you must anticipate an "adrenaline dump,"and train for it accordingly.

Overcoming an adrenaline dump quickly is critically important. If you don't train for such a scenario, the chances of the adrenaline dump hindering your movements and thinking increase dramatically. However, if you anticipate this expected effect and practice for it during your functional workout sessions, you not only improve your fitness level−you increase your chances of survival. That's why the following drills are so practical.

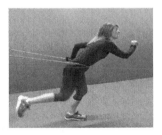

Band running can be done indoors or outside.

Adrenaline-Dump Drills (with bonus cardio and calorie-burning benefits)

Band-Running—If you're grabbed really quick and you're startled, your heart is going to race. One practical drill you can start practicing is running in place with a band around your waist while your partner securely holds the band behind you. Drill this for one minute, running as fast as you can. Then move immediately to a functional fitness drill that requires practical self defense motions. This trains you to move quickly and mimics the fast-breathing, adrenalin-pumping, and heart-pounding you may encounter in survival situations.

Run-Abs-Claw-Punch—Place a band around your waist and have your partner hold it securely behind you. Begin to run forward, with your partner holding on to the band without allowing you to move forward very much. You'll essentially be running in place with tension for 10-15 seconds. As soon as you stop, immediately get into a sit-up position on the floor. Your heart will be racing. Have your partner hold a medicine ball or a striking shield at your eye level and begin to do a sit-up while you punch or claw the ball with your hands or fists. You're essentially doing a sit up while hitting the ball at the same time, and continue to punch or claw as you move back down. This is a tremendous workout for the core and the triceps. You'll get a very challenging workout as you train these functional moves, all while mimicking the heart-pounding scenario of an adrenaline dump.

Run-Abs-Claw-Punch Drill

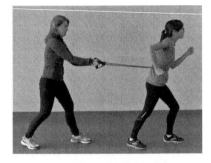

Place a band around your waist and have your partner hold it securely behind you. Begin to run forward, with your partner holding on to the band without allowing you to move forward very much. You'll essentially be running in place with tension for 10-15 seconds.

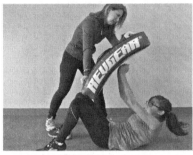

As soon as you stop, immediately get into a sit-up position on the floor. Your heart will be racing. Have your partner hold a medicine ball or a striking shield at your eye level and begin to do a sit-up while you punch or claw the ball with your hands or fists.

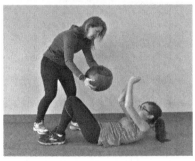

You're essentially doing a sit up while hitting the ball at the same time, and continue to punch or claw as you move back down.

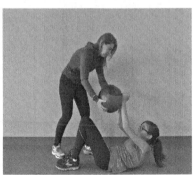

You'll get a very challenging workout as you train these functional moves, all while mimicking the heart-pounding scenario of an adrenaline dump.

Jab-Cross-Sprint—Begin in a comfortable boxing style stance with one leg forward and with your body angled. Bring your hands up and keep them relaxed in front of you. Jab with your front hand (eye jab) and cross punch or jab the pad with the opposite hand immediately as your front hand travels back to its starting position. Immediately sprint 25 yards past your partner and sprint back. Switch legs and repeat on the opposite side. Work up to practicing on each side about 10 times. If you're in a location that allows you to practice your powerful yell without others getting concerned, feel free to use it when you execute your strikes.

Hit-Hit Side-Shuffle Squat—Begin in a comfortable boxing style stance with one leg forward and with your body angled. Have your partner hold a hitting pad or medicine ball in front of you, at about your eye level or slightly higher. Hit the target twice with your forward hand as fast as you can, then side shuffle away, squat, and side shuffle back. Repeat with the opposite side. Work up to 10 repetitions on both sides. This is an intense series of movements that will tax your cardiovascular system very quickly. Take your time with this drill initially and gradually increase the speed, force of your blows, and the intensity.

Pushups

When you push someone away, what does that motion look like? If you thought of a pushup while being upright, you're absolutely correct. This is why pushups should be on your list of functional fitness allies. Pushups are an absolute must and there's simply no getting around them —unless you have a physical limitation that prevents you from performing them or similar motions. In such cases, other drills can be performed, such as throwing and catching a lighter medicine ball while sitting or laying down.

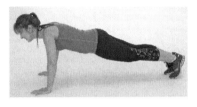

Pushups can be done just about anywhere and require no equipment.

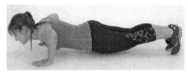

The ability to perform a forward striking motion with some force is very important. This can throw an assailant off balance and buy you valuable time to escape or perform an effective offensive attack. Forget about "girl" pushups where you place your knees on the floor to help you up. If you can't do a full pushup yet, begin training for the movement on a raised surface such as a bench or table, or against the wall, working up to the floor. Another way to build up to doing a full pushup is by holding a plank. Simply get into a pushup position where your body is away from the floor and hold there as long as you can. Slowly work on one push up, focusing on good form as your strength increases. In time, you'll easily accomplish 10 full pushups, and you can then graduate to doing "knuckle" planks. That simply means you'll make a fist like you're punching the floor and rest your weight on both fists while holding a plank. You should feel your core working when you work on planks, along with your arms. Finish the plank when you feel you can't hold good form anymore or if your back starts to bother you. Eventually, you'll be able to do knuckle pushups. Imagine that!

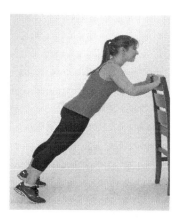

If doing a full push up is too difficult initially, start against a wall or a sturdy chair (placed solidly against a wall to avoid moviement) and continue to practice until your strength increases.

Fitness Band Motions

There are countless drills that can be done with fitness bands. Your body does not know if you're lifting steel barbells, a can of refried beans, or pulling on a challenging fitness band—all it knows is that there's resistance it must overcome to perform a motion. A key area where many individuals can definitely get stronger is their back. This is where pulling motions come into play to strengthen these often underutilized muscles.

Standing Band Jab-Cross—Some very practical band motions for self defense include the "jab-cross" with the band. Performing this drill challenges and strengthens the triceps and chest muscles. You simultaneously benefit by practicing functional movements that train you to deliver an effective blow to the face. Simply hook the band around your back or have a partner hold the band behind you. Grab the handles and jab (punch forward with your lead hand), then cross (retreat your lead hand and extend your rear hand while shifting your hips enough to reach the target) while holding the resistance of the band with each hand. The jab will look like a forward punch and the cross will be delivered with the opposite hand toward the same target. Feel the resistance the band provides and, if necessary, adjust the tension to allow for the full extension of your arm (leaving just a slight bend). Work up to 10 repetitions on each side. If the motions feel too easy, increase the tension in the band by stepping forward or get a thicker band. Be sure the band comes back to the starting position slowly, without snapping back.

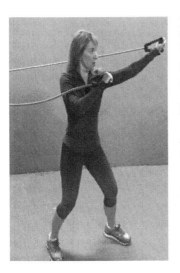 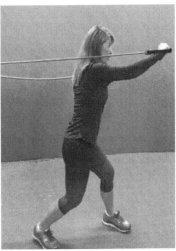

Jab and cross with resistance bands. Keep visualizing your assailant as you perform your fitness drills.

Band Jab-Cross Backward-Shuffle—This is a practical drill to add to your functional fitness routine because it trains movements most individuals don't commonly engage in such as moving backwards. It also builds strength and stamina. Jab-cross using the band that's wrapped around your back, then back-shuffle quickly for about 7-10 steps (you can choose to drop the band or hold on to it as you shuffle back), and run back to your starting position. Practicing drills where you shuffle backwards is practical because it allows you to keep your eyes on the assailant after you strike him. When you gain enough distance you can turn around and run. This avoids turning around too soon, when an attacker may not be sufficiently incapacitated and goes to grab for your hair, yanking you backwards. The back-shuffle allows you to gain your distance and gauge if the aggressor is incapacitated enough for you to run to safety.

Medicine Balls

One of the challenges with cardiovascular exercise machines such as treadmills and elliptical trainers is that they're don't sufficiently build your upper body and bone density. That means that if you fall on your arm, you could break it if your bones are frail. This is why it's a good idea to practice arm-impact training every day.

Medicine balls are incredibly versatile for practicing functional movements, especially those that build arm bone density. Every time a ball hits your hands when it's caught, you're stimulating your bones to build bone density, similar to the leg bone-enhancing benefits attained from running.

Medicine Ball Squat and Press—A good motion to practice to push someone away is the squat, leap, and press with a medicine ball. This develops core strength and explosive ability. Begin by standing tall with a medicine ball in front of you. Pick up the medicine ball and hold it in front of your body. Now squat, then leap into the air while simultaneously pressing the medicine ball in front of you. Feel the challenge in your arms and legs. Work up to 10 repetitions. This drill is practical in that it mimics your position of squatting down and standing up (you can imagine that you're quickly getting off the ground or chair) as you push someone away with explosive power.

Medicine Ball Knees—Begin by facing your partner and have them gently toss the medicine ball toward your knee. Knee the ball with the top of your knee, connecting towards the center of the ball if possible. Pretend you're a soccer player. Alternate knees. Note what it feels like to connect your knee with an object. It feels vastly different from connecting your knee with just the air. If you don't have a partner to work with, you can start by dropping the ball on your knee and kneeing the ball forward away from you. The key with this drill is to develop the ability to get your foot off the ground quickly. Getting your foot off the ground quickly and kneeing accurately (as developed by this drill) will help you knee a target of your choice on an assailant.

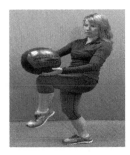 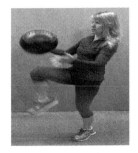

Medicine Ball Elbows—Begin by facing your partner and have them gently throw the medicine ball towards your upper body, preferably above your shoulders. Lift your elbow and angle it to the side, parallel with the floor. The knuckles of your arm will be facing the ceiling. Imagine that you're balancing a cup of water on your extended elbow. As the medicine ball nears your elbow, tense your arm and elbow the ball back to your partner. Breathe out as you hit the ball. Work toward rotating your waist and core, really putting some energy into the elbow hit. Note how it feels to hit something with your elbow. Practice the motion in the air during the day to develop good form. Practicing elbowing an object such as the medicine ball or a solid pad also helps to build bone density.

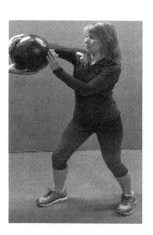 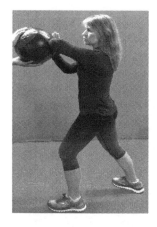

Balance and Sensitivity Drills

Few fitness routines incorporate balance drills, yet this type of training is very important for your fall and injury prevention, cognitive stimulation, and over-all health. In a confrontation, you may be pushed or pulled off balance, making quick equilibrium recovery a critical skill. One fall to the ground may mean breaking a limb or loosing consciousness if you hit your head. This is why balance training is so important.

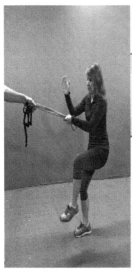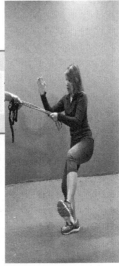

Have your partner hold a fitness band or towel at one end while you hold the other. Stand on one foot. Have your partner try to pull you off balance from side to side while you try to maintain your body upright in a stable position.

As you begin to test yourself by challenging your balance, your body learns to react faster and more efficiently to being unstable. Balance training helps you control your center of gravity and increases your movement efficiency. There are many balance challenging devices, from the Bosu balance trainer to Si-boards, and even thick ropes placed on the floor. Since you never know the nature of the surface you may be standing on when you're called to respond to a confrontation, it's a good idea to train on different surfaces such as sand, concrete, and grass.

Partner Forearm Sensitivity and Balance Drill—Face your partner and place your forearm against theirs. You will both have just extended your "bridge." Now try to pull each other off balance with the connecting arm. Take turns. These movements develop the back and the core. You also learn peripheral perception (where you are in space). See if you can get a good grip on your partners arm and pull them into an eye jab or a throat strike. Try pulling them into your elbow. This is a fun drill that's functional. To add the element of balance to this drill, simply stand on one leg. Remember to alternate legs and note which side feels more stable.

The Squat-and-Kick—You can attain a functionally strong gluteus by practicing a squat and a kick. Simply squat with your legs apart and as you come up to stand, kick forward with one of your legs. Pretend that you are kicking someone in a valuable target. This is a more advanced drill that develops balance, coordination, and explosive strength. The movements also build your gluteus muscles.

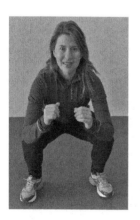

1. Start by standing up, then squat.

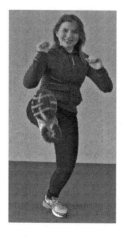

2. As you get up, use your balance to kick with one of your feet. Be sure to alternate your feet.

Be sure to practice the concepts you learned in this chapter and share them with your children and others who may benefit from the knowledge. Practicing functional fitness is practical and can be fun–especially when you feel empowered because you know that what you're doing may help you in a situation that counts.

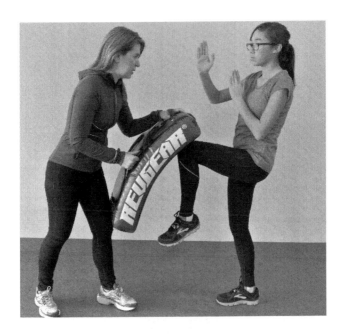

Chapter 10

Safety Away from Home

Chances are great that you have to drive, commute, or travel to get to work, school, grocery stores, appointments, sporting events, concerts, and to visit family and friends. That essentially means that you spend at least some of your time in a vehicle of some sort on the road; either as a driver or a passenger. Traveling may also require that you stay in hotel rooms, other peoples houses, and that you have to unexpectedly camp-out at the airport or train terminal if your mode of transportation is delayed or cancelled.

Sure, that's all part of modern living today, but it should also give you more reasons to think about your safety away from home in a variety of expected and unexpected situations. For example: driving a car, walking to and from the car, and even getting in and out of the car can lead to personal safety challenges that need to be addressed; and using public bathrooms that are remote and open to anyone may also pose a danger. Additionally, it's important to remember that when you're in any foreign environment—which can be a warehouse next to your house, a country that you've never visited, or a neighborhood you know very little about—you have virtually no control of that environment, including the kind of people you share it with. Luckily, you do have control over yourself.

In this chapter, we'll look at some common on-the-road and travel scenarios, with the goal of expanding your awareness and safety when you're away from home. Of course, every potentially challenging situation that you may encounter cannot be encompassed here; some of the topics are so vast they can take up a whole book in themselves. So it's best to spend time thinking about where you'll be ahead of time and focus on what you may need to bring with you, along with the most favorable actions you can take to decrease your risk of harm or, at the very least, increase your comfort level if you're stranded. The following information will give you some ideas to build on.

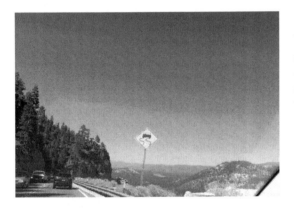

You may spend time in a vehicle of some sort on the road.

Consider Various Road Situations Ahead of Time

It almost goes without saying that you should know where you're heading off to and have detailed directions of how to get there if you've never been to your destination or if you're thinking about traveling to an unfamiliar area. Don't count completely on your cellphone, GPS device, or your memory and personal navigation skills; while all are convenient and important, they (and you) can sometimes make mistakes; and satellite reception can give out at any time, leaving you wondering where in the world (literally) you are. It certainly doesn't hurt to print out driving directions ahead of time and highlight your map with your destination routes beforehand to have as backups.

One thing that most people lack in their car is a good set of maps. Maps of your immediate environment, along with maps of the surrounding areas and the destination that you're traveling to (if it's far) should be front and center on your list of important car items (a lengthy list is provide later in the chapter). Many tourist centers and sometimes AAA offices will often have free maps; and even if they don't, it's well worth it to invest in good maps and route books available at most book stores to have on hand in all your vehicles, and one for home use too. Take the time to study your maps, learning the roads in your vicinity and the places where you're traveling to and from to familiarize yourself with the areas in the event of unexpected road or bridge closures and if you get lost, miss an exit, and other emergencies that may come up such as running out of gas (not uncommon).

Many emergency road situations can be complex because of the countless variables that you will have to contend with—and those variables can change by the hour, minute, or second. You may start out stranded with a stalled car on a heavily trafficked road during the day, which can suddenly become increasingly desolate as night approaches. Your car can break down on a clear summer day only to have heavy rainfall come down on you two hours later. So the point to consider here is that a number of variables will change your decision about what to do from moment to moment. The goal should be to think ahead and use your imagination to come up with many possible scenarios and see what can improve your safety in those scenarios ahead of time; be it having certain items with you, taking specific actions, or (ideally) both.

It's obvious that if you get a flat tire in the middle of the busy highway during rush-hour in the morning and make a quick call to your towing company, they'll likely be able to assist you relatively quickly. If that's the case, be sure to alert others of your exact location (your spouse, friend, relative) and stay inside your car (if it's safe) with the doors locked until the tow truck arrives. However, when other variables are added to that situation, the decisions that you have to make may become less obvious.

For example, imagine that you still have that flat tire in the middle of the busy highway during rush-hour in the morning but this time you realize that your cell phone is out of battery or you forgot it at home. What's your next move? It will all depend on a number of variables: How well do you know the area? How close are you to an exit? Will walking to that exit put you in greater danger? If you're close to an exit that has businesses or a gas station from which you can make your phone calls, are you capable of walking there wearing the shoes you have on? Are they high-heeled shoes that you use only during work because you don't have to walk much? Do you have a spare pair of flats or sneakers in your trunk for these kinds of situations? If it's not safe to get out of your car for whatever reason, do you have a pen and paper to make a quick sign that says: "Need, help, Call 911," or "Call for assistance," to place against your car window and alert other drivers to call for you? This can sometimes put you in greater danger because it tells highway predators that you're stranded and no one is on their way to help you.

So you see, there are countless factors involved in making the most practical decisions that you can during less than perfect situations, and the goal is for you to think about how to best deal with those scenarios ahead of time.

Doing so prepares your mindset and allows you to anticipate what you may need to have with you to make life safer and more pleasant. Because you'll want as much assistance as you can get when you're away from everything that's familiar to you.

Be Aware of Highway Predators

Roads, particularly desolate highways, can put anyone in a vulnerable situation very quickly; one of the reasons being is that today's highway predators and other criminal opportunists have their eyes peeled on desolate highways looking for their lucky break, namely: you and your family. Logistically speaking, they have the perfect opportunity to commit their crimes because many secluded roads are ready-made "crime scene number 2" locations; without people around and plenty of camouflage-like terrain to hide them and you from prying eyes and ears. Those reasons alone should make driving a *premeditated though-process* on your end before you even get into your car.

The first thing to understand about your vehicle is that it's not a sealed fortress. Your car windows can be easily broken, making it simple for an aggressor to come inside or quickly drag you out into the nearby secluded bushes or his own automobile. Even without breaking the windows, today's criminals have access to and practice with various tools that make opening a car door a quick breeze; which they may choose to do if they want to use or sell your car, or to avoid leaving telltale signs of forced-entry.

It's important to also point out (as mentioned previously) that all predators–including highway predators

−can look like the average person, i.e. *anyone*. They can seem car-savvy, friendly, charming, and act like your best buddy. They can dish out a good act of care and concern, lulling you into a false state of comfort; the kind that makes you breathe out a sigh of relief and thank the heavens that your super hero arrived just in time to save the day. He most likely didn't.

Understand that when people feel vulnerable and need assistance, that's the time they usually start to let their guard down because of desperation and panic. They begin to give away their power to others, especially when it comes to making decisions. It seems easier to let someone else−anyone who seems to know better−take over; putting you back into that infant-like state when your parents kept you safe from harm. Highway predators know this. They also count on your natural tendency to trust the goodness you expect to find in others, especially when you're in trouble. Since people tend to project on to others the qualities they posses themselves, honest and trustworthy individuals often assume that other people are that way too; something that all predators use to their advantage.

So if you're stranded in your vehicle (without the possibility of your car exploding, drowning, or other danger that requires immediate evacuation), don't be too quick to exit your car and greet strangers with hugs and handshakes who pull over to check out your situation; especially if you're in a high traffic area. Instead, be extra alert and aware.

If you see someone approach your car, be cautious rather than trusting. Remember, trust must be earned so why automatically give that trust away to someone who allegedly offers you assistance? If you get a bad vibe, keep the doors locked and tell or motion to the person that help is on the way. Make it sound like someone is about to arrive really soon. You can show your cell phone (they won't know the battery is dead) and motion that you've already called for assistance and someone (your husband, brother-in law, towing company, friend who just finished teaching a boxing class) is on their way to help you.

If the potential highway predator motions that there's no reception in the area, it could be an indication that he's testing your response. You can say that your car has an auto-emergency system (if it doesn't look like an antique model vehicle) and that they've already confirmed your location and sent out for help. If that's not an option because your car simply looks too old or decrepit, you can say that your brother, spouse, or carload of friends are only a short distance behind you on the road and will be passing you momentarily; you'll catch a ride with them. Remember, you don't own any stranger (especially when you're in a disadvantageous situation) your honesty or politeness. Try to give off a confident and relaxed vibe, as if help is really right around the corner.

Be aware that the highway predator may get back into his car and wait to see if someone actually arrives to help you; or he may drive away and come back a short time later to see if you're still there. If you see him do this, it's obviously a bad sign that he has you on his radar and intends to wait things out. Without question, this is a bad scenario for you as the highway predator is actively escalating the situation; but at least you're aware and alert enough to know where you stand so you can begin to take the next step.

That next step may mean taking more drastic actions if your options are very limited. It may be getting dark and the passing traffic may be getting slim. You may be running out of choices and may consider quickly evacuating your vehicle to flag down an incoming motorist. Of course, that will alert the highway predator that you're desperate, but at least it will be in the presence of other people rather than in seclusion. If you can, at least grab a makeshift weapon of some sort in your car; a pen, heavy flashlight, umbrella, or anything else that can give you the edge if you're physically accosted by the highway predator.

Sometimes waiting inside the car is not the best option. If your car breaks down at night by a more lighted area, head for an open business with lights if it seems safer than waiting for a highway predator to come upon you. But if your car stalls in the middle of nowhere at night, consider exiting your vehicle and walking to hide yourself in an area (like the bushes) where you will not be seen by other cars. Sure, it's scary to walk through uneven, possibly wet terrain in the dark, but that's certainly safer than waiting for a potential highway predator. At least you won't be trapped inside the car. That's one of the reasons that having a blanket, flashlight, snack foods, and makeshift weapons can come in so handy. You can use the blanket to sit on or to keep you warm. A flashlight can be used to help you see and to temporarily blind a potential predator who may approach you in the dark. Makeshift weapons can help give you the equalizer you need against an attacker; and it's certainly easier to wait things out with snacks on hand than on an empty stomach.

If you decide to hide away from your car, do your best to keep a visual on it. You may see others stop by and check it out. The best case scenario would be for law enforcement or highway patrol to stop and look your car over. That could be your opportunity to flag them down for assistance, keeping in mind that they may see you as a potential threat too. Anyone suddenly emerging from a hiding spot can seem suspect, so approach with your hands up where they can be easily seen (without holding anything remotely dangerous looking) and address them in a polite manner. At that point, you'll likely get the assistance you need to call others who can help you and get a ride to a safer location (the local police station or another safe waiting spot).

However, sometimes opportunistic thieves or predators stop to get a closer look at your vehicle for diabolical reasons: like stealing your car, tires, rims, or anything else they think is of value inside. If you see someone break your car window while you're hiding safely out of sight, it's a good indication that the person want's the car or what's in the car. Thankfully, that won't be you.

Tourist Opportunists

Traveling can be fun and educational, but only if your safety comes first.

When you find yourself in an unfamiliar neighborhood or area, whether in your own country of residence or another continent that you've never been to before, you essentially become a kind of tourist; which can have it's own set of safety challenges for several important reasons.

The first is that you don't know the area well, which means you can get lost very quickly and find yourself in places where you don't necessarily want to be—like the backyard of the neighborhood drug dealer or a local prostitution house. Less than savory neighborhoods tend to have numerous criminal elements, who can locate you quickly and understand your vulnerability. Many have little to lose by robbing you or worse.

It's not uncommon to get into a kind of tourist "bubble" and start to believe that you're immune from harm just because "you're visiting." You may think that your awkwardness and lack of directional skills will inspire others to help you simply because that's what you'd do in a similar situation; which can lead you to turn over your trust too easily.

Tourist opportunists *are* on the lookout to help—it's just that they're on the lookout to *help themselves*; to your belongings, your body, and sometimes your children. So when you're lost and disoriented in any unfamiliar environment, be cautious about advertising that fact to play down your vulnerability. Remain calm, confident, and in control. Cautiously and selectively decide the best business to ask directions. Obviously a gas station is preferable to a liquor store, and a grocery store is preferable to a bar. Use your common sense and intuition before you approach anyone for assistance.

The second challenge is that you often stick out like a sore thumb compared to the rest of the local population. You look different, you dress different, you act different, you walk different, you give off a different vibe, and you may speak a different language or have a distinct accent even if you speak the same language.

Both of these reasons make you extra vulnerable (and invaluable) to tourist opportunists who are on the lookout for easy targets loaded with money, jewelry, and credit cards. These criminals know you don't travel without any means, so they see you as the perfect candidate to rip off, rob, or worse. They can see you coming a mile away and they do have some advantages that you don't: they know the in's and out's of the area; they have access to criminal buddy's who can assist them; and they know if law enforcement will pose a threat to them or not.

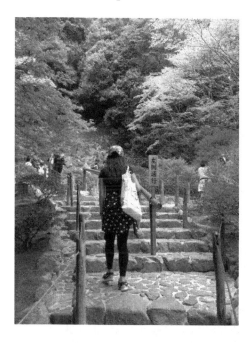

Traveling can be fun and educational, but only if your safety comes first.

Local criminals will often screen you and watch to see how you operate. Are you traveling alone? Are you with other locals they're acquainted with or have seen around often? That can change their game plan because it means that other people who "know what's up" are looking out for you. Are you with a local tour group? That also offers some advantages because your tour guides will often share critical safety information that you may not know otherwise. Tour companies also try to maintain their image for business purposes so they'll often go out of their way to make sure they don't put you in undue danger.

The key with traveling is to try to blend in as much as you can. That means you must do your research about where you're going. Read blogs with peoples experiences about where you plan to visit; search for videos of the area to see what you can expect ahead of time and familiarize yourself with how people dress and carry themselves. Are there plenty of people just like you visiting the place? Do you know local people who live there? Will they show you around? Use common sense and don't advertise your jewelry or display a full wallet to others. You never know who's watching but you can assume tourist opportunists are.

It's also a good idea to travel with other trusted people who are safety conscious. The individuals in your travel group can look out for each other and notice when things are amiss. You'll also have a wider range of personalities who have different skills and talents that can come in handy in challenging situations. It can also be more fun to explore new areas in a group setting.

If you travel with others, discuss a backup plan of where to meet should someone get separated from the group. Make sure everyone is wearing a watch and mark the time and location you'll meet up if people decide to explore the vicinity on their own. Have a plan of what to do and where to go if an individual is missing or becomes ill or injured. It's always preferable to be prepared in advance rather than try to figure out what to do when every second counts.

Generally, it's not a good idea to bring your precious and irreplaceable items with you when you travel. Leave them at home. It's too easy for luggage to get lost so a good rule of thumb is to only take possessions with you that you're prepared to leave behind permanently without being too upset. Also, be extremely cautious about getting into taxis or accepting rides from individuals you don't know. Consider researching reputable shuttle companies for transportation and always leave a copy of your itinerary with friends or relatives so at least someone knows what area you plan to be in and how to locate you.

If you carry your identification with you, consider making a few copies of your passport, drivers license, etc., to keep at home and to give to a trusted friend or relative to have on file. If your identification is lost or stolen when you're on the road, at least you'll have a way for your friend to email or fax you a copy of your identification, which can be helpful especially in foreign countries where you may need an embassy to assist you with getting back home. It certainly does not hurt to have copies of important documentation if you should need them in the future.

Carjacking Aggressors

Do you get into your car when you're distracted by texting, talking on the phone, or adjusting your purse? The more preoccupied you are around your car or as you're getting in your car, the more vulnerable you become to car aggressors.

Carjackings can happen very quickly, particularly at road intersections, parking lots, and driveways. Some carjackers work as part of a team and ambush an individual from both sides of the car.

Generally, there are a few basic goals that an aggressor has when he confronts you near or in your vehicle: The first is that he want's only your car. He may ask for the keys outright or he may threaten you with a weapon while demanding your car keys. If you're outside your car and no one is inside your vehicle (like your child), can you quickly throw the keys his way while you take off in the opposite direction? If the answer is yes and he goes for the keys to get your car, consider yourself lucky. Head to a safe location on the side of the road that's harder for him to attempt to run you over. Giving a car thief your car quickly and having him drive away is the best case scenario considering you didn't get injured—you can always replace a car.

The second goal is much more dangerous because the assailant is interested in you. If you didn't check the inside of your car before you got in it, an attacker may be hiding in the back seat. Similarly, if you didn't lock your car immediately when you got in it, an aggressor can slip in right next to you, often with a weapon. Being held up at gun or knife point is one of the last things anyone expects, which is the reason most individuals don't know how to respond.

You may become trapped in your car with an assailant who holds a weapon to you and shouts out instructions for you to drive. You may not know where you're headed but you understand that it won't be a good place for you. That's why, in such a tough situation, some experts suggest that you consider crashing your car. Yes, it seems counterintuitive and you do run the risk of injury, but at that point your options may be severely limited. If you decide to crash your vehicle and the aggressor is in the front seat next to you, try to aim the car to crash into an object that's closest to him and furthest from you. If it's a pole, stop light, or sign post, aim the car to hit your passenger side. Obviously, you will damage the object you hit along with your car—but you may increase the chances of escaping with your life.

The noise, commotion, and attention from an accident gets people on their phone, and some individuals even stop to check if people are hurt. Some experts suggest that crashing the car may be your only chance of escape. Yes, you may have to deal with fines for damaged property, increased insurance premiums, and the hassle of getting a new or used car, but what's the alternative?

Understand that whether you or the aggressor is driving the car, you're headed to "crime scene number 2." Your options are very limited. Are you going to jump out of a moving vehicle and risk death? Are you going to scream and yell inside the car where only the aggressor can hear you? Crashing the vehicle may be the only choice that gives you a better chance. It's possible that you may be wearing a seatbelt and he isn't, in which case there may be a greater chance of you getting less injured than him.

Forget about driving around and looking for something ideal to hit, the perfect target is not likely to appear. Don't waste time by analyzing if it's cheaper to hit a trash can or the stop sign; time is imperative so if you decide to crash the car, create as much noise and commotion as you can with crashing your vehicle (do your best not to hit innocent pedestrians). If you're in the passenger seat, assume that he's driving you to crime scene number 2, so if your hands are free do your best to gouge the aggressors eyes and force him to crash the car any way that you can.

The third goal of the aggressor is to take the car, along with you and possibly your child. Sadly, some women have been carjacked with their children still in the car, and others have been pushed out of the vehicle only to see it being driven away with their child inside.

One of the most important actions you can take if you drive your children around is to talk to them in a matter-of-fact way about the possibility of a carjacking. Keep in mind the age and emotional makeup of your child when bringing up the topic. Explain that it's important that they respond to your commands should a situation arise so they don't become paralyzed. If you tell them to get out of the car quickly and run they need to be able to do that with lightning speed. This is especially critical if you get into a physical struggle with a carjacker. It's possible that during a carjacking scenario you won't be able to help your kids, so they must know ahead of time that they need to listen to your commands and quickly respond to them. That alone may save their life. Educate them in advance that even if they see you being hurt, they still need to work hard to save themselves. Of course it's not a pleasant topic to bring up but it's a worthy one; there's a lot at stake—your kids.

Public Bathrooms

Public bathrooms can be some of the most dangerous places you'll ever find yourself in. When you see the "men" or "women" sign or drawing outside of a public bathroom, what do you think stops the men from going into the women's bathroom and vice-versa? Actually...nothing. That's right, signs are not a guarantee that someone will follow them. In some ways, signs almost give us a false sense of comfort. We start to believe that just because a sign says something that everyone will follow it's command. But we know that's not reality because people ignore signs all the time; just think of a Stop sign and how many people run right through it when driving.

Public bathrooms in remote areas won't have many people around, and some will have poor lighting, and plenty of spaces for attackers to hide undetected–both singularly and in groups. That's why public bathrooms should be high on your radar of dangerous locations. They can quickly become a ready-made "crime scene number 2" setting for an attacker looking for a target.

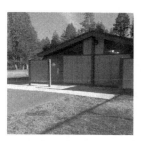

When you see the "men" or "women" sign or drawing outside of a public bathroom, what do you think stops the men from going into the women's bathroom and vice-versa? Actually...nothing.

How easy is it for an assailant to walk into a secluded bathroom when no one is around, get into a private stall, close the door, and step on the toilet so no one can see him if they look underneath? It's a breeze. All he has to do is wait for a good opportunity to attack. The flimsy "locks" on bathroom stalls are more for decoration that for safety. A two year old can push most open without much effort. An assailant can also crawl underneath the stalls, which tend to have enough space for just about any size individual to crawl under, to attack when you're in a vulnerable position. Some unsuspecting women have even had photos and videos taken of them while going to the bathroom by predators who used small cameras that can be positioned underneath the stall. You may have read of these instances in the media.

If you absolutely must use a public bathroom, consider if the location is well placed within a busy area such as an airport terminal that has security cameras outside and a constant flow of people coming in and out. Compare this with a secluded bathroom in a park that has absolutely no security and is in a remote location where others can't see or hear you.

If you decide to go in, do so with extreme caution. Assume that one or several predators may be inside or hiding in a stall. Peek in the bathroom to see if anything is out of order before you fully commit to going in. Obvious signs are men's legs in a stall. Check if the doors to the stalls are open and if anyone is inside. Sure, it takes a few extra seconds to do this, but at least if there is someone hiding, you'll be in a better position to respond or flee than if you were sitting or squatting on the toilet with your garments pulled down.

Having a friend with you is helpful as the person can stay right outside the bathroom door while you're inside. At least someone will know where you are and will keep an eye out for anyone who may enter after you're inside. They can also glance into the bathroom ahead of time with you to make sure that no one is visibly hiding in a stall.

If you enter an empty bathroom and go inside a stall, keep your eyes and ears open for anyone who comes in and for any unusual movements (like a predator who's checking to see who's inside a stall rather than a woman who comes in to use the bathroom). Take care of your business quickly, wash your hands if it's safe, and leave without lingering to check your hair, makeup, or text messages. The less time you spend handing around inside the better.

You never want to be trapped in any closed space in a remote location, which public bathrooms sometimes are.

Avoid talking on the phone or texting near the toilet. You'd be surprised how common it is for a cell phone to accidentally find it's way into the toilet bowl. Keep your cell phone close but not close enough to fall in and become useless because it's been immersed in water.

Some women who travel frequently on the road keep a personal makeshift port-a-potty in their car. This can be a simple plastic jar with a wide opening that's lined with a trash bag. While far from glamorous, in emergency situations, a makeshift port-a-potty may sometimes be a safer option than venturing outside the vehicle.

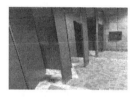 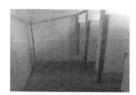

Public bathrooms in remote areas won't have many people around, and some will have poor lighting, and plenty of spaces for attackers to hide undetected—both singularly and in groups.

Common Sense Road Advice

- **Avoid parking next to a van or truck**—Because highway predators often work in teams, a van or truck can hide numerous assailants inside. The size of a van also makes visibility difficult and blocks both your car and you from the view of others. People can't readily see what's inside a van, which make them extremely dangerous in kidnapping scenarios. Be extra alert around vans, trucks, and mobile homes. Keep your distance and be prepared to escape if necessary.

- **Don't get out of your car if you don't feel safe**–Be extremely cautious if your car gets "bumped" while you're at a signal or a stop sign in a poorly lit, secluded location. Keep your car doors locked, window up, engine running, and call the police immediately. If the person steps out of the rear vehicle and asks you to come out, signal for them to follow you to another well lit location (preferably a busy grocery store parking lot or police station). It's a good idea to have a 3x5 card already written out with your insurance information and a general contact number that you can slip through the crack of your window to hand to them if they start pressing you for the information. If you feel afraid, say so, and ask them to follow you to the nearest well-lit convenience store. A normal person should have no problem with such a request–*but a predator will*. Those who insist that you get out of your car should be viewed as extremely dangerous. Don't be afraid to drive away if you feel threatened in any way. If you're asked why you left the scene of the accident, feel free to state that you were scared for your life.

- **Be weary of offers for help**–If you're riding your bicycle and get bumped by a car, be weary of the driver who offers to drive you to the hospital. The same goes for a person who lightly hits your car and offers to drive you to the hospital. Don't get into another persons car under any circumstances. Keep your cell phone handy and call the police. The chapters in a later section of this book will discuss items that can be carried on your person or in your bag that can provide additional assistance and support.

Helpful Car Contents

With all the time that you and your children may spend in your car, it's imperative that you keep it in good working order. Be diligent about keeping the tires inflated, the oil changed, and the battery in good standing. Make it a habit to always keep your doors locked and the windows rolled up more than half way.

It's a good idea to keep your vehicle's gas tank at least half-full always, instead of allowing it to get close to empty. Sure, you'll have to fill up sooner, but what's the additional inconvenience compared with the knowing that you have plenty of gas to get you to a more secure location should you have to drive away from a dangerous situation?

It should be noted here that, while you can get away with keeping your home space messy or cluttered, doing the same with your car can spell disaster. You can't afford to be scouring around for maps, flashlights, and other essential items that you may need at a moments notice under piles of food wrappers, dirty laundry, discarded facial tissues, and other odds and ends that simply don't belong in a car. Remember, a car is a relatively small space, so the amount of practical items that you can fit in there is severely limited. That's why you want to make the space counts and that can only be created by a clean and orderly interior.

Take time out of your schedule to spend on cleaning out your car. Get several large garbage bags ready and clear out everything that you have in your car into them, including all the stuff that's between and under the seats. You can go through this stuff in the comfort of your home later. Vacuum and dust the interior. With all the time that you probably spend in your car, you'll want to create healthier breathing conditions, without excessive dust and grime that can add to allergies.

Once everything is vacuumed, cleaned, and dusted, it makes sense to store items in your car that will assist you in an emergency. Consider keeping the following items in your car; along with anything else that may be relevant to your unique situation:

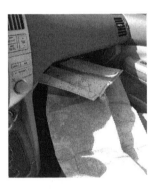

Maps–It's a good idea to have maps in your car. Keep them close and handy, not buried under piles of stuff and hard to get to.

Cell phone and car charger (most newer cars can charge a phone with the proper charger)–You should ideally keep your phone in your purse so it travels with you everywhere, and keep your purse down and away from sight of people passing by your car. A cell phone is particularly imperative if you're stranded on a secluded road; although you must be prepared for the possibility that you will not have reception, or your phone may unexpectedly break.

Quality Flashlight (with additional batteries)–A good flashlight can help you see in the dark if you need to start walking. You can also use it to signal to others your location. A flashlight is not helpful if the batteries are dead. Test your flashlight weekly or monthly and keep additional batteries in the car in case the primary ones die out.

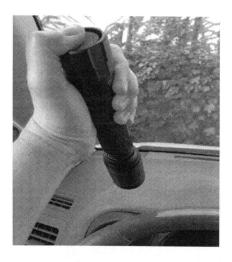

A quality flashlight can help you see in the dark and may also be used as a makeshift weapon.

Jacket, hat, gloves, and long pants–You never know when or where your car might stall and how long you will need to wait for assistance. That's why it's a good idea to have a set of extra clothing in your car. At the very least, keep a pair of long pants, a jacket, a hat, and a pair of gloves or mittens. These items can mean the difference between being warm and dry or cold and miserable as you wait for help to arrive. It's also a good idea to keep additional clothes for your children.

Sneakers or comfortable shoes for walking long distances–If you're on your way home from a party and you're wearing shoes with high heels, consider carrying flats with you. Keep a pair of sneakers in your car so that if it stalls and you need to walk to safety you'll be able to without a problem. Walking long distances in high heels can prove to be disastrous; they'll slow you down and may damage your feet. In a situation where you're far away from home, you'll be happy to have comfortable footwear that allows you to quickly get to a safe location with the least amount of discomfort.

Bottled water–It's always a good idea to keep various sizes of bottled water in your car. If you're stranded in the heat, you and your family can stay hydrated; avoiding dangerous dehydration. If you have kids, it's even more imperative that they stay well hydrated. Water is critical for your car too, so if it suddenly overheats, you can use it to cool the engine (if you know how). You may also unexpectedly run out of window-wiper fluid and may need to add water so you can spray down the windows to see well. Be sure to rotate your water stores to keep the water fresh and check that it does not evaporate in the heat after time.

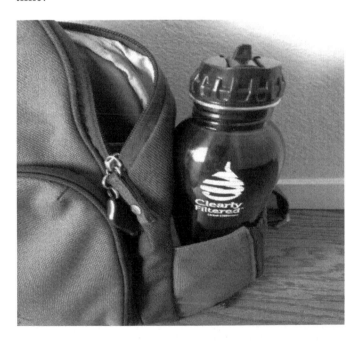

It's practical to keep a water bottle that has a quality built-in filter with you in the car or on the go. You can quickly fill up with water from any faucet and have clean water to drink. The Clearly Filtered steel water bottle with built-in filter shown here is available at clearlyfiltered.com.

- **Nutrition bars**—Nutritional bars are small and easy to store. Most can last for over a year, and when eaten provide quick energy if you and your children suddenly become stranded. It's certainly more pleasant to wait for assistance when you and your kids are less famished; it also provides needed calories and extra energy to keep your brain fueled for clearer thinking.

- **Blankets**—Keeping a few light blankets or long sheets is very helpful when you must wait for help away from the car. Blankets can be used to sit on rough terrain or to keep you and your kids warm during the cold weather. They can also be thrown over overhead branches to provide shade in hot weather. Cozy blankets give children a sense of comfort if they're stranded with you in the car, which helps to keep everyone more relaxed.

- **Cards with road assistance and emergency numbers** —When you're under pressure in a stranded situation, your memory may not perform as well as you're used to. That's why having a few easily accessible cards with emergency numbers are critical. Cards provide you with correct numbers in the event you suddenly lose your memory—a common occurrence in stressful situations. They're also handy to take with you to a public location if you need to use a public phone when your's is out of battery or broken. Most of us rely on our cell phone to hold all our contact numbers but if the phone is lost or broken we have no access to those numbers. This is where the cards come in. Keep several in your car and one in your purse and let your kids know where they're located so they can call for assistance if you're injured or unconscious.

- **Facial Tissue**—Facial tissue can come in handy when you run out of toilet paper. It can be used to blow your nose when you have allergies or colds as you drive. Who want's to drive with a runny nose and no facial tissue? It can also be used to wipe unexpected spills, clean your windshield, and wipe your glasses. The uses are endless.

Use Extra Caution in Hotels

Hotels, motels, bed-and-breakfast facilities, rental cottages, and other away-from-home locations could pose additional safety dangers that you need to be aware of. The main one is *accessibility*.

When you get the key to the place where you're staying, *who has the other key*? Potentially...anyone. Housekeepers have keys, door attendant's have keys, hotel and condo management have keys—and their friends, relatives, acquaintances, and paying predators can easily get those keys too. So when you lock the door of your rented space, you essentially don't do much for your safety because *anyone* can have a key that allows them access. Thankfully, there are some preventive measures you can take to help make staying in locations away from home safer.

First: Avoid demonstrating that you're traveling alone. If you're in the hallway getting in or out of your room and notice someone around, say something like: "Honey, I'm back," or "I'll be back soon." Let those around you think that there's a man in the room waiting for you. When you leave the rented space for a short time, allow the TV to stay on so it sounds like someone else is in the room.

Second: Check the room thoroughly for anyone hiding in the closet, bathroom, and under the bed when you first enter. Predators love to hide-in-waiting because they know that most people don't check their room. They can pop-out when you're at you're most vulnerable: getting out of the shower, sleeping, or undressing.

Third: Prop a chair against the door after you've searched it so you're alerted if it opens, and consider investing in a door alarm, both for travel, and for home use. A door alarm is very handy for travel or for those who live alone. Unfortunately, many assaults take place in hotels and similar locations away from home. By placing an alarm under the door—when it opens—the door will press on the alarm and it will exude a loud screech. The wedge shape of the alarm also makes it more difficult to open the door.

Predators always want the element of surprise to be in their favor. They count on shocking their target and are often unprepared to hear a blaring alarm, especially in hospitality locations they're familiar with. Loud noises bring attention from others, who often try to figure out what's going on. Since predators don't want attention, witnesses, and potential rescuers, they'll often flee when presented with alarms.

A door alarm is also handy to keep under your desk at work as it can be pressed at any time with your foot when you feel threatened. Several can be used in the same location: one under the main entrance, an additional one under the bedroom door, and one next to your bed. The more noise created, the better.

Clothes and Shoes for Outside-wear

There are many appealing outfits that some women enjoy wearing to attract men; unfortunately, those outfits also make them look more desirable to predators too. That's why it's critically important to give your outside wear careful consideration.

Sure, within the safe sanctuary of your own home, you can get away with wearing fuzzy slippers, six-inch heels, and clothing so tight that you have to hop instead of walk to the kitchen. You can tune-out to your hearts desire and completely relax your guard. You can crank up your music and walk around while texting, singing, and vacuuming all at the same time. But should you do all that outside your door?

In the real world, you may want to wear comfortable shoes that you can easily run in; stable footwear that allows you to move quickly from side to side and backwards if you need to. High heels that you can barely walk in and tight skirts or pants that you can't effectively kick in may signal "easy target" to a predator. Ask yourself, *are the benefits worth the risk?*

When you wear a constricting, tight-fitting outfit and high heels, how fast can you escape from a predator? If you were forced to run for your life and your high heel got caught on something, will your changes of falling to the ground increase or decrease?

Consider that the items that you are wearing may be used against you. A thin scarf or a necklace may turn into a choking weapon. Items that women don't commonly think of as potential hazards include pierced ears; dangling earrings can be grabbed and yanked so hard that they cut through the lower fleshy part of the ear lobe; causing tremendous pain. Rings can get caught on objects with fingers being twisted and stuck.

The idea is to provide very little ammunition against yourself to a predator, and to use all of his weaknesses to your advantage.

Useful Products for the Road and Home

There are certain products that can be invaluable assets to give you an extra "edge" by increasing your visibility, supplying loud noises, and offering "hand-extensions" that save your hands from injury. Take a look at the following products and consider incorporating them into your safety routine both on the road and at home if applicable.

Tail-Cap Flashlight—Our eyesight is very poor in the dark because we're not nocturnal creatures. That's why having a tail-cap flashlight is an absolute necessity—it increases your visibility and allows you to gauge a situation from a safer distance. The difference between a regular flashlight and one with a tail-cap is the on-off button at the end. This distinguishing feature is especially helpful when you're getting in and out of your car during the evening or in poorly lit parking lots or stairways.

When approaching your car at night, have the car keys and tail-cap flashlight in your hand—it serves no benefit hiding in your purse. Turn on the flashlight and look under, around, and in the car's front and back seats *before* getting in (anyone can buy a gadget that opens a car door in seconds).

Holding the flashlight with the fingers around it and thumb at the end is an offensive posture which prepares you to strike at an instant or blind an assailant in the dark, causing them to lose their night vision and buying you time to get to safety.

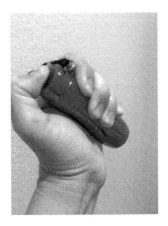

When approaching your car at night, have the car keys and tail-cap flashlight in your hand.

Body Alarm–A body alarm is a very practical device that can be clipped on to a purse or belt. If you're in a threatening situation, simply pull the pin. The assailant will be bombarded with a loud, ear-piercing noise that he's not going to want to be around. Carry the body alarm with you always. If you have a car alarm, have your hand on the panic button when approaching the vehicle. If your car is parked close enough to your home, keep your car key next to your bed so you can press it quickly to sound the alarm and wake up the neighborhood.

Practical Key Chains–There are a number of practical key chain options available that can give you the "edge" in the event of an attack. The "key" is to have them handy, always in your hands, and know how to use them. The Kitty Kat Key Guard, developed and designed by renowned actress/ martial artist and women's advocate, Spice Williams-Crosby, is designed to look like a friendly cat. The shape allows your hands to easily grip the key chain and the ears are designed to light up anyone's nerve center to let go. It is an item of opportunity to be used to make space in the event of an attack. If you intend to use your key chains for self defense purposes, practice doing so in advance, and continue to train with them often.

This key chain can be ordered from ifightformylife.com.

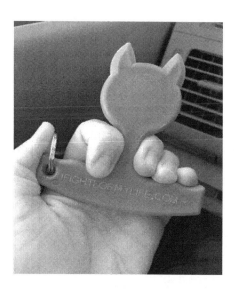

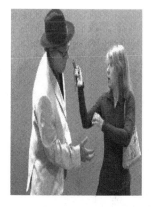

Door Barricades—Door barricades help keep someone from coming through your door quickly, no matter what they do with the locks and even if they break the frame. Heavy gage, specially flanged steel lag bolts go into your 2X4 jack studs and an incredibly strong, square tubular steel bar prevents the door from opening. When you want to go out, you simply lift the barricade off of the bolts and set it to the side. When you're inside, you slide the bar on to the mounts. Installing a door barricade usually takes less than 5 minutes. Door barricade companies can be found in the resource section of this book.

Door Brace—For a very small monetary investment, you can purchase a door brace that makes it much more difficult to force your door open. Door braces are portable and allow you to move them easily from one door to another. You simply place the brace under your door knob while the opposite end rests on the floor and resists sliding. Some door braces have varying size slots that allow you to collapse the brace and take it with you while you travel. These are practical for hotel rooms and other places where you want to reinforce your door.

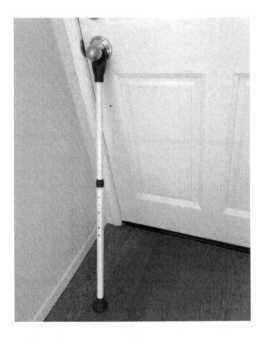

A door brace makes it much more difficult to force your door open. It's also portable and can be used when traveling.

Door-Wedge Alarm—A door-wedge alarm looks very much like the rubber stoppers you use to prop doors open, except when you put one in place and turn it on, if someone tries to open the door, the pressure on top of the door wedge will trigger an internal loud alarm to go off. That causes a lot of noise; not something that criminals want.

Door-wedge alarms are inexpensive and portable, making them ideal for hotel rooms, college dorms, or even to keep under your desk at work. If you have one under your desk, you can simply press your foot on top of it to set off the loud noise.

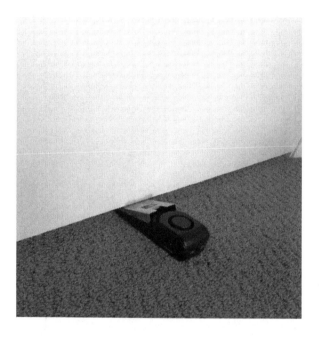

Door-wedge alarms are inexpensive and portable, making them ideal for hotel rooms, college dorms, or to keep under your desk at work.

Chapter 11

Step Into Your Power

It's empowering to take charge of your life. Being in control of your thoughts, beliefs, emotions, body, and actions empowers and liberates–you feel as if you can do almost anything!

We are all born innately powerful. Unfortunately, with the repressive programming that society plants in many of us, it can be a challenge to reclaim, develop, and become comfortable with our own power.

It's important to note that just because you make the choice to empower yourself, does not mean that you disempower someone else. Remember, empowerment benefits everyone.

Control Stress

We can only "spin so many plates" at a time. Once we get beyond our threshold, something is going to fall. So given that we can only spin so many plates, lets make sure the ones that we are monitoring are the most important because if we keep adding unimportant plates, then we're not going to be able to maintain the important ones. The more plates we add the more stress we're under.

That's why stress is one of the most debilitating things in life. Stress increases our levels of cortisol, a stress hormone that is released from the adrenal glands. Cortisol eats away a portion of our brain called the hippocampus, which is responsible for memory and creativity. The more stress we are under, the more we start to lose our mental faculties.

Tips to Manage Stress

- Take a walk around your neighborhood (if it's safe), or drive to a pleasant and well populated area where you can walk to clear your mind.

- Incorporate relaxation techniques into your daily routine to keep stress in check. Consider yoga, tai chi, gentle stretching, or use a foam roller to release tension.

- Become conscious of your breathing patterns during the day and notice when you tend to hold your breath. Practice deep diaphragmatic breathing throughout the day. Slow, deep breathing delivers more oxygen to the brain and the rest of the body.

- Enjoy a warm and soothing lavender Ebson salt bath to help relax the muscles and induce more relaxation.

- Take care of yourself by investing in quality body care products that contain organic ingredients. Look for products that are bottled in glass rather than petroleum-based plastics to avoid applying bottle-leaching petro-chemicals to your skin. Read labels carefully and support companies who don't test on animals and who go out of their way to operate with the utmost respect for human rights, animal rights, and the environment.

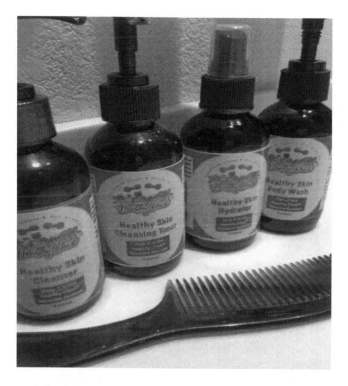

Healthy Chick organic body care products can be found at healthychick.com.

- Consider meditation practice. This is simply focused attention, often directed at the breath or a mental image. When you keep your focus in one place, you stop harboring on anxious thoughts and the constant mental chatter that often fills the mind. Meditation can quiet the mind and help release stress.

- Consider nutritional support to help with stress. The B vitamins, Siberian ginseng, ashwaganda, shizandra, vitamin C, and phosphatidylserine can help control high cortisol levels.

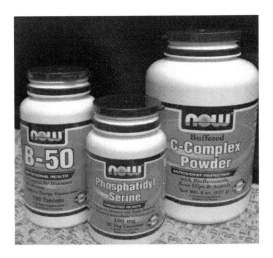

- Eat a nutrient filled plant based diet brimming with antioxidants and phytonutrients to assist with stress. Consider incorporating a nutritional product called Earth (available from HealthForce Naturals) to help with grounding and nutrient support.

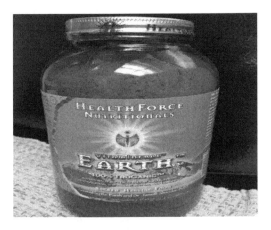

Earth from HealthForce Naturals.

Take Charge of Your Finances

When you take control of your finances, you gain confidence, independence, and peace of mind. While single women often have an individual bank account as part of their lifestyle, sometimes, when they get together with a partner, they open a joint account and close their individual one. However, some experts believe it's a good idea for both parties to keep their own accounts, particularly women. Any good man would not have a problem with his significant-other having an account of her own.

If a man is in charge of all the cash in the household, what happens if he's suddenly violent to the woman living with him and possibly to her children? How many options of quick escape are open to her without money? But if she has her own finances, there are many more choices available. Money can buy the airline or bus tickets that can put a safe distance between a woman and a violent man; and it can buy food, shelter, and much more. That's why it's a good idea for women to educate themselves about money as part of their empowerment.

Some experts urge individuals to consider maintaining an individual bank account; an account that only you have access to. You can add a beneficiary or a Power of Attorney to your account (check with your legal and/or financial adviser about what's best in your individual situation).

Should you tell the man in your life that you have such an account? That's up to you. The key point is that he does not have access, because if he does—he can close the account at any time, even without your knowledge. Also, it's wise to ask yourself some important questions, namely: Will he ask you for extra money when he's short on funds?

Will he expect you to spend the money in your individual account for expenses you both previously shared, essentially siphoning the money out of your account through other methods? If the answer is yes, it may not be a good idea.

If you're looking to escape from a man, saving money can help with the getaway–if that's the case, you'll probably want to keep the account hidden. Most financial institutions offer online statements at account opening (check with your financial institution). This means that you will not receive paper statements but you can view them online. If you file taxes together with a man but you want to keep your special account hidden from him, consider keeping your funds in a non-interest bearing account so that a 1099 will not be generated at the end of the year (interest earnings over $10.00 generate a 1099), so he's not alerted. Again, check with your tax advisor about your individual situation.

Is having an individual bank account a good idea for a married woman? Many experts think so. Remember, just because people are happily married today does not mean that things will stay that way indefinitely. It's wonderful to think positive and hope for the best, but it certainly hurts no one for you to have your own account should things change in your future. A woman must have some financial means of independence should the man she's with suddenly morph into a predator. This has happened in the past to countless women so it's crucial that you have the financial means to get out quickly. In a violent situation–it can mean the difference between life and death.

Releasing an Abusive Shopping-Affair

Industries that specialize in the selling of goods know that women are the most profitable consumers because they frequently do most of the shopping. This is one of the reasons manufacturers have turned shopping into an elaborate affair–as a new mode of fun "recreation," igniting a "shop until you drop" mentality that can easily spiral into an addiction.

We all have things that trigger a different "high" in us. Since we're all different and unique, we get excited and motivated by different things. For a shopping addict, the thrill or "high" is from the purchase instead of from eating a box of cookies, for example.

Shopping has been touted as a fun time that fills the empty void in life and it offers another distraction to the dissatisfaction and discontent we may feel (similar to processed foods). So it comes as no surprise that countless women today consider themselves to be "shopaholics."

A shopping addiction, just like any addiction, is disempowering because we don't have full control of our actions. Instead, our brain is hijacked by the "high" we experience, in spite of it having a negative affect on us and others.

Like many addictions, excessive compulsive shopping for stuff that's not needed and generally not even wanted later, often leads women into financial trouble and a cluttered house. Shopping becomes a game of finding something that will fill the void of the emptiness that's felt inside, and just like any addictive behavior, excessive shopping leads to guilt, shame, fear, and worry. Many of the items bought are frequently not even used or needed, adding to the frustration of others who share the home and have to live with the additional clutter.

It's often easy to spot a shopping addict–just visit their house. While they may have lovely and unique items, it's sometimes difficult to even distinguish many of them under the other stuff that's laying over them. The closet of a shopping addict may be crammed or spilling over with clothes and shoes that still have price tags; many in original boxes. Their closet can be filled with clothes they've never even worn or used once and abandoned.

As with all addictions, healing a shopping obsession takes awareness, time, and plenty of self love. It's a compulsive behavior that needs assistance and understanding. A shopping addiction is nothing to be ashamed of. We've simply been "hooked" by our brain chemistry to respond to a habit or pattern that lights up certain pathways in our brain to create "feel good" chemicals. A shopping addict is no different.

Take a look at the following suggestions in healing a shopping addiction and don't be afraid to seek professional help.

• Take honest inventory of your closet space. Weed out items that you have not worn for 1 year. Chances are you will not wear them again. Donate the items to a local charity. Keep the donation receipts for your records.

• If you feel compelled to shop because it's your only form of recreation, consider joining a class or club that meets during your favorite shopping hours. Hold yourself accountable for attending your new workshop.

- Consider leaving your credit cards at home and only carry enough cash to pay for immediate expenses. When the urge to purchase something that you don't need comes up, you'll have to make a trip home to pick up the cards, which may diminish the "rush."

- Take an objective look at your home. Are there piles of "stuff" everywhere? Do you have a difficult time finding anything? Sometimes de-cluttering your space can be very healing and recharging. Make a commitment to stop buying more items at least until you clean, organize, or donate unnecessary stuff from your home.

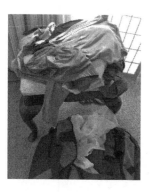

Take an objective look at your home. Are there piles of "stuff" everywhere?

- Have a yard sale. Place price tags on everything you don't need and invite your friends and neighbors to your yard sale. Your clutter can be something that someone else desperately needs but can't afford. You also help the earth by recycling the items since they do not end up in a landfill.

- Check out library books about organizing, clearing clutter, or feng shui for ideas and inspiration to keep your personal space nurturing, welcoming, and a healing place where you can recharge and rejuvenate your sprit. Victoria Moran's book *Shelter for the Spirit* is a good choice.

- Seek professional help or a support group where others share their successes and provide a supportive environment for healing a shopping addiction.

Empowering Your Space

If you avoid cleaning and organizing your living space, it can become stagnant and cluttered, sapping you of energy and enthusiasm. Messes that are not dealt with can be draining since we're constantly looking at them when we're home because they call for our attention; so we frequently ignore them because we don't want to deal with the unpleasant task of cleaning or organizing.

Just like any disempowering habit that can escalate over time into a full-blown problem, clutter has a way of accumulating in the home if it's not kept in check.

Clearing clutter from your living environment can be very empowering and emotionally cleansing. Take a look at the following suggestions for clearing up your personal space.

- Take a slow look around every room in your home. Start with a small area if you're pressed for time, perhaps just the top of your desk. Look at the items it's holding. Are there photos which bring back bittersweet memories that make you frown or feel bad? Replace them with photos that lift you up. Are there files that you're avoiding filing? File them now. After you finish one area and see how great it makes the surrounding space look and feel, you'll be further inspired to continue with the rest of the room. As one room is finished, gradually work toward other rooms, including closets.

- Is there a thick coat of dust on your tables, bookshelves, or stands? Start to think of house chores as your special time to get in touch with clearing out the unnecessary grime out of your life. Envision that you're clearing any negative energy that you may be feeling every time you dust.

- Make cleaning a workout. Squat while you pick up items off the floor, feeling the stretch. Reach with each arm as you stretch to dust higher shelves. Twist and bend using your legs as you lift items. Try to use your non-dominant hand when vacuuming, sweeping, or mopping to engage another part of your body, activating your cognitive function and improving your balance.

- Remember that the tidier your living space is, the less risk you and others have of tripping and falling. You're essentially also making your space safer when you clear clutter.

- Removing unnecessary objects also allows more space in a room and promotes oxygen circulation. Regular dusting keeps allergies at bay, since you inhale what's in your environment.

- Beautify your living space with items and decorations that lift you up and remind you of good times. Consider posting collages and affirmations in key areas where you will see them often.

Creating Your "Empowerment Toolbox"

There are many empowering "tools" that can encourage self esteem, confidence, and vitality. One method of putting these helpful modalities to use involves creating your own unique "empowerment toolbox."

Think of your empowerment toolbox as a holder that contains useful personal assistants that give you a helping hand when you need them. The tools in your empowerment toolbox are always available to aid you and you have complete choice about which ones you want to use.

The following partial list of empowering tools are supportive companions to have in your empowerment toolbox and you can always create additional collaborators that are unique to your needs.

Your Power Collage—When we read a long and detailed description of an item, it gives us a good idea of what it looks like, but seeing a picture of that item instantaneously conveys the information to us easily, without any need for words, because pictures can instantly communicate with our mind.

Naturally, the fashion, fitness, and diet industries use this knowledge to their full advantage to sell more products. Unfortunately, most of the images they disperse are unrealistic and disempower women in ways already discussed in earlier chapters. Thankfully, there's a powerful tool that we can add to our "empowerment toolbox" that can help counter the negative programming dispersed by these industries. It's called a Power Collage.

Sometimes our visions are too vague or we may have a difficult time trying to picture what it is that we really want. A Power Collage allows us to see our goals and aspirations immediately and at any time. When professional race-car drivers experience a blowout and their car steers them into a wall, they're trained to turn their face and look towards where they want to be heading—away from the damaging wall and back on the road towards their goal. A Power Collage similarly encompasses the same mental framework. It focuses our vision in the direction we want to go—keeping us on the right tract. A Power Collage is like having your own personal coach around you 24 hours a day, motivating and inspiring you continually. Your Power Collage should be updated as often as you like so it's just like you—a work in progress.

As a child, you may have worked on making a collage during art class in school, but if not, know that it's an easy process. Simply take a sheet of paper or a piece of cardboard and attach photos, drawings, affirmations, or a combination of all these to it. Choose images that raise your self esteem, motivation, and creativity. If a photo of a woman boxing inspires you to feel empowered, attach that image to your Power Collage. If you want to eat more whole unprocessed foods, including a photo of colorful fruits and vegetables will serve as a good reminder. You have absolutely free reign about what to attach to your collage, so choose content that makes you feel happy and uplifted. Keep in mind that a Power Collage should inspire and motivate, not make you feel bad about yourself. Some women enjoy adding their own affirmations such as: "I'm healthy, powerful, and filled with vitality." Choose words and images that assist with your empowerment and experiment with making more than one Power Collage to post on the fridge, in the bathroom, next to your bed, and even a tiny miniaturize size one to keep in your purse or wallet.

Your Self-Reflecting Journal– A personal journal can act as a window to self knowledge. The simple act of writing can have an immense affect on your psychological, emotional, and physical health. One of the most powerful ways you can assert control over your life is by keeping a personal journal. Writing down thoughts and feelings allows you to express yourself and release stress, helping you to feel better.

Your journal allows you to observe any patterns, cycles, and trends that you may be experiencing. Sometimes, just becoming conscious of your habits allows you to make a better decision about keeping or changing them. A journal does not have to cost much and you can use any notebook. Simply allow yourself some time to write in a comfortable location whatever comes to your mind. It's also a good idea to date your entries for future reflections, seeing how far you've come in your self empowerment journey.

Connecting with Nature–In the past, we spent most of our time in nature. Today, many people barely get a drop of sun on their skin. The closest some individuals come to seeing a plant is on a travel magazine.

Simply going outside and taking a walk in nature with a friend or alone (if it's safe) can rejuvenate and uplift emotions and put a smile on our face. Scenic views inspire self reflection and contemplation; important qualities that open up a dialogue with the self.

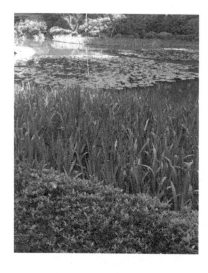

Embracing and reconnecting with nature can be one of the most healing and nurturing activities we can engage in.

If you live in the city and are not surrounded by much nature, try to bring some healthy living plants into your home and office. Plants provide oxygen, help clean the air, release positive energy, decrease stress and electronic radiation, and help with relaxation. If you can't have plants for various reasons, bring in photos or drawings of nature, sculptures that remind you of nature, or pictures of trees and flowers. You can even make a personal nature collage. If you're cooped up indoors all day, try to get outside often.

One of the best activities for optimal health is spending time outdoors. Getting fresh air and exposure to greenery is calming and recharging. When our skin is exposed to sunlight, it produces vitamin D (a hormone). Vitamin D helps in calcium absorption and is also imperative for normal immune system function.

Your Buying Power–You have tremendous buying power. This is one of the reasons advertising companies work so diligently in influencing you toward their products. When you make a purchase, you cast a vote with your money by telling both the store and the manufacturer to keep carrying and producing that item.

Since every dollar you spend casts a vote for the raw materials that were used to make that product, it's important to avoid supporting companies that are harmful to our health and the planet. Paying for organic produce keeps organic farmers in business and buying Fair Trade products keeps companies more accountable to their workers. Purchasing cruelty-free cosmetics and beauty care items ensures that their ingredients were not painfully tested on innocent animals. When you bring your own bags to stores, you also stop harmful plastics from ending up in our landfills and oceans. Remember that every purchase you make is a vote, so cast it wisely for those items that will empower both you, your environment, and future generations.

Make Five Minutes for Positive Change–Taking a few minutes daily or weekly to get involved and speaking up for what's important to you can greatly assist your wellbeing. Every minute spent on a worthy cause helps those in need and makes you feel good. Being active and involved in clubs or groups that work toward a beneficial cause is empowering. Taking a few minutes a couple of times per day to fill out a petition about a topic that you feel strongly about is often a doable and pleasant activity that empowers and motivates. You take an action that directly helps others, which is healing to everyone involved. Start an online blog, make videos, and write articles about worthy causes that stir your spirit into action. Consider signing the 5 Minute Activism petitions on the www.johnpierre.com website.

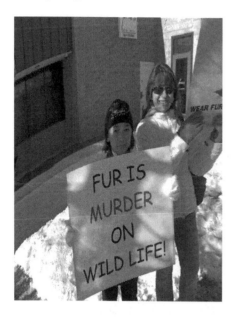

Every minute spent on a worthy cause helps those in need and makes you feel good. Being active and involved in clubs or groups that work toward a beneficial cause is empowering.

Build a Social Connection—Positive, recharging, and supportive social ties can be powerful motivators and stress reducers. Consider joining a dance club that combines social interaction with physical activity and the mental challenge of learning new dance steps. Spend time with people who make you feel happier and more lively. Explore joining a walking or biking club or try yoga or whole foods cooking classes. Volunteer in your community or help someone in need.

Express Yourself: Love, Laugh, Play—What do you enjoy doing? Is it writing, painting, making music, or dancing? Having fun, laughing, and playing are basic biological drives that are integral to our health and wellbeing, similar to restful sleep and healthy food.

We are designed to flourish through play during our lifetime. Play is natures most advance process for promoting brain development and social integration. It energizes, enlivens, and helps ease stress. Our best memories are often of playing (think vacation) and making play a part of our daily lives is one of the most important factors in being happy.

Sadly, as we age, we're told to work harder, impress the boss, and make more money, leaving little time and energy for playing. But when we put play aside, we begin to suffer from bad moods and the inability to experience sustained pleasure. Play promotes creation of new connections between neurons which are important and essential to continued brain organization. So remember to bring the important element of play into your day often.

There are many modalities that can encompass your "empowerment tool box." Consider adding essential oils, massage, and your own personal creative modalities and ideas to your empowerment toolbox, and share them with others.

Invite in Gratitude

Taking a few minutes in your day to be grateful for something is one of the most beneficial actions you can take to improve the quality of your life. Gratefulness cultivates mindfulness and keeps you focused on a positive aspect that you appreciate. That does not have to be grandiose. Being grateful increases optimism because you validate that there is something positive in your life. It also reduces stress and focuses your vision on the positive. It encourages a more positive outlook and teaches you to be aware of the good that you already have.

Remember to use the words "Thank You" often. Regardless of what your current challenges hold, it's important to pause often to appreciate all that you have. When you "count your blessings," and give thanks for them, you allow yourself to enjoy them. A good way to instantly boost your mood is by making a list of everything in your life that you feel grateful for. Keep adding to the list as you think of more ideas. You can look at your "gratitude" list in the morning, evening, or anytime during the day.

Your Gratitude List: What are you grateful for?

- My vision
- My hearing
- My teeth
- My ability to walk
- My sibling
- My sense of humor
- My home
- My work
- The list can go on indefinitely...

End of the Day Reflections

A powerful way to end the day is by reflecting on your thoughts, feelings, and actions of what transpired. This helps you to commit to doing even better tomorrow. Consider asking yourself questions that allow you to honestly reflect about your day and think of ways you can continue to improve. This will increase your overall life satisfaction and happiness.

- What made me the most happy today?

- How can I increase my happiness tomorrow?

- In what ways did I help others today?

- How did I assist in helping the planet today?

- Did I stay true to my morals and values?

- Did I follow through with my goals today?

- What actions did I take today to increase my family's safety?

Remember to encourage yourself, give yourself positive feedback and use the information found in this book to increase your safety and empowerment.

Afterword

This book has asked you to think in new ways regarding your safety. It brought up topics for your consideration related to your awareness, health, and mental and physical skills. The overriding goal has been to increase your chances of survival in adverse situations.

It is the authors sincere hope that these writings inspire you to increase your self esteem and self worth—to empower all aspects of yourself. Because when you care about yourself, you won't allow others to demean or disempower you. When you love yourself, you'll take actions that increase and affirm your invaluable self worth.

Be strong, be savvy, and stay safe.

Resources

Books

The 4-Ingredient Vegan, by Maribeth Abrams and Anne Dinshah

21-Day Weight Loss Kickstart, by Neal D. Barnard, M.D.

The 22 Day Revolution, by Marco Borges

The 30-Day Vegan Challenge, by Colleen Patrick-Goudreau

The 80/10/10 Diet, by Dr. Douglas N. Graham

Absorb What is Useful, by Dan Inosanto

Becoming Raw, by Brenda Davis, R.D., and Vesanto Melina, M.S., R.D., with Rynn Berry

Becoming Vegan, by Brenda Davis, R.D., and Vesanto Melina, M.S., R.D.

Breaking the Food Seduction, by Neal D. Barnard M.D.

The China Study, by T. Collin Cambell and Thomas M. Cambell

Compassion: The Ultimate Ethic, by Victoria Moran

The Complete Idiot's Guide to Plant-Based Nutrition, by Julieanna Hever, M.S., R.D., C.P.T.

Defeating Diabetes, by Brenda Davis, R.D., and Tom Barnard, M.D.

Disease-Proof Your Child, by Joel Fuhrman, M. D.

Eat and Run, by Scott Jurek

Eat Vegan on $4 a Day, by Ellen Jaffe Jones

The Engine 2 Diet, by Rip Esselstyn

Farm Sanctuary, by Gene Baur

Finding Ultra, by Rich Roll

Fit Quickies, by Lani Muelrath

Foods for the Gods, by Rynn Berry

Forks Over Knives, by Del Sroufe, with Isa Chandra Moskowitz

The Happy Herbivore, by Lindsay S. Nixon

Healing the Vegan Way, by Mark Reinfeld

Health Can Be Harmless, by H. Jay Dinshah

Here's Harmlessness, by H. Jay Dinshah

How Not to Die, by Michael Greger, M.D., with Gene Stone

How to spot a dangerous man before you get involved, by Sandra L. Brown, M.A.

The Lean, by Kathy Freston

The Love-Powered Diet, by Victoria Moran

Mad Cowboy, by Howard F. Lyman

Main Street Vegan, by Victoria Moran

The McDougall Plan, by John A. McDougall, M.D., and Mary A. McDougall

McDougall's Medicine, by John A. McDougall, M.D.

The Most Noble Diet, by George Eisman, R.D.

My Beef with Meat, by Rip Esselstyn

My Body Is My Own, by Ty Ritter

Out of the Jungle, by H. Jay Dinshah

Peace Pilgrim, by Peace Pilgrim

The Pillars of Health, by John Pierre

The Plantpower Way, by Rich Roll and Julie Piatt

The Pleasure Trap, by Douglas J. Lisle, Ph.D., and Alan Goldhamer, D.C.

Prevent and Reverse Heart Disease, by Caldwell B. Esselstyn, Jr., M.D.

Shred It!, by Robert Cheeke

Strong on Defense, by Stanford Strong.

Super Immunity, by Joel Fuhrman, M. D.

Thrive, by Brendan Brazier

Thrive Fitness, by Brendan Brazier

Tao of Jeet Kune Do, by Bruce Lee

Uncooking with Jameth and Kim, by Jameth Sheridan, N.D., and Kim Sheridan, N.D.

Unprocessed, by Chef AJ, with Glen Merzer

Vegan Bodybuilding & Fitness, by Robert Cheeke

The Vegan Diet as Chronic Disease Prevention, by Kerrie K. Saunders, Ph.D.

Vegan for Life, by Jack Norris, R.D., and Virginia Messina, M.P.H., R.D.

The Veggie Queen, by Jill Nussinow, M.S., R.D.

Whitewash, by Joseph Keon

Whole, by T. Collin Campbell, Ph.D., with Howard Jacobson, Ph.D.

The World Peace Diet, by Will Tuttle, Ph.D.

DVDs

Calorie Density, by Jeff Novick, MS, RD, LD, LN

Digestion Made Easy, by Michael Klaper, M. D.

Don't Mess with M.A.M.A. Mothers Against Malicious Acts.

Earthlings, by Shaun Monson

Forks Over Knives, by Lee Fulkerson

From Oil to Nuts, by Jeff Novick, MS, RD, LD, LN

Sense and Nonsense in Nutrition, by Michael Klaper, M. D.

Unity, by Shaun Monson

Websites

www.allisonsgourmet.com —organic vegan treats

http://www.bar-ricade.com/ – Door barricades and more

www.compassioncircle.com – dedicated to creating awareness and expanding compassion toward all beings with who we share this planet.

www.cok.net – Compassion Over Killing: non-profit animal rights organization

www.chefrobertsdirect.com—Matt's Munchies, organic premium fruit snacks

www.doctorfood.org – Dr. Kerrie Saunders: nutritional and emotional support

www.doctorklaper.com/index.html – Dr. Michael Klaper: plant based-information and videos

www.drbronner.com – quality toothpaste, soaps, and more

www.eatunprocessed.com – Chef AJ: whole-food recipes and information

www.enerhealthbotanicals.com—quality nutritional support and more

www.evohemp.com —Nutrition food bars

www.farmsanctuary.org – Farm Sanctuary: non-profit organization and sanctuary for farm animals

www.farmusa.org – non-profit organization dedicated to animal rights, newsletter, nutritional information, and more

www.freethegirls.org – Free The Girls non-profit organization works to provided jobs to survivors of sex trafficking in developing countries.

www.healthforce.com – Dr. Jameth Sheridan: health and nutrition information, podcasts

www.healthychick.com – Dr. Kim Sheridan: fitness, organic body-care products, and more http://ifightformylife.com/−Spice Williams-Crosby: women's self defense and empowerment

http://www.jarrettarthur.com/blog/−Jarrett Arthur: customized self-defense for women.

www.jaykordich.com − Jay Kordich, The Father of Juicing: juicers, newsletter and more

www.jeffnovick.com − Jeff Novick, MS, RD, LD, LN: health and nutrition information

www.johnpierre.com − John Pierre: articles, recipes, and links

www.livingwithharmony.org − John Pierre's animal sanctuary and retreat center

www.mainstreetvegan.net − Victoria Moran: nutritional information and more

www.mamaselfdefense.com−Mothers Against Malicious Acts. Jarrett Arthur website for women's self defense.

www.marcpro.com − Marc Pro devices for muscle recovery and performance

www.mercyforanimals.org − Mercy for Animals: non-profit organization devoted to animal rights and compassion

www.mikemahler.com − Mike Mahler: fitness articles and podcasts

www.miyokoskitchen.com − quality plant based cheese-like spreads

www.neilmed.com−quality nasal care products and more

www.nutritionfacts.org − Dr. Michael Greger, M.D.: nutritional information, videos, and more

www.newgy.com−quality robo-pong accessories and equipment

www.pamelaandersonfoundation.org − Pamela Anderson: supports organizations and idividuals that stand on the front lines in the protection of human, animal, and environmental rights.

www.thepatriotnurse.com/-Practical information on medical preparedness, and more.

www.peta.org –People for the Ethical Treatment of Animals: dedicated to animal rights education and more

www.pcrm.org – Physicians Committee for Responsible Medicine website with resources and nutritional information

www.projectchildsave.com – Ty Ritter: nonprofit organization dedicated to helping prevent child abductions and kidnapping through education and public awareness campaigns

www.revolar.com– portable device that alerts others in an emergency at the press of a button

www.seashepherd.org – Sea Shepherd: non-profit organization dedicated to saving marine life, raising awareness, and more

www.Si-boards.com – quality balance boards

www.simplydara.com – organic raw plant based snacks

www.sproutman.com – quality sprouting products and information

www.tonyblauer.com– Tony Blauer: practical self defense information

http://transitionsglobal.org/–Transitions provides comprehensive restorative aftercare for girls rescued from sex trafficking.

www.twinbunnies.com – Barbie Twins: animal rights information and awareness

ourrescue.org – non profit organization dedicated to rescuing kidnapped children from slavery.

www.veganfusion.com – Chef Mark Reinfeld: plant based recipes and more

www.veganoutreach.org – nutritional information, newsletter, and more

www.vegsource.com – health and nutritional information, articles, videos, and more

www.waterbrick.org– delivery and storage system for people in need of bulk water and more

www.woodstocksanctuary.org – Woodstock Farm Sanctuary; non -profit organization for the protection of animals www.yummyplants.com – Rebecca Gilbert: plant based nutrition information, resources, and much more

www.12minutekitchen.com – easy plant based recipes and cooking ideas

Companies

Blendtec – quality blenders; available at www.johnpierre.com: click Shop, Blendtec

Boku – superfoods, tea, plant-based protein powder, bokusuperfood.com

Brooks Running – brooksrunning.com, quality sportwear, shoes, and more. Special thanks to Brooks for suppying the garments worn for the photo shoots.

Clearly Filtered – clearlyfiltered.com, quality water filters for home or on the go.

Do Terra – www.mydoterra.com/johnpierre – quality essential oils.

Dynamax – quality weighted balls, www.medicineballs.com

The Fanciful Fox – quality vegan soap and candle company, www.fancifulfox.com

Flexi-Bar – Information on Flexi-Bar and more, flexi-bar.com/us/en/home

Floracopeia – quality essential oils; available at floracopeia.com

Florax DS – pribiotics for improved digestive health; available at www.florax-ds.com

GoodBelly – organic digestive helpers; available at www.goodbelly.com

Happy Tiffin – stainless-steel containers for food storage; available at www.johnpierre.com: click Shop, Happy Tiffin

HealthForce Nutritionals – quality green powders, protein powders, and a wide variety of nutritional supplements; available at www.johnpierre.com: click Shop, HealthForce

Herb Pharm – quality herbal products, www.herb-pharm.com

Instant Pot– quality pressure cookers, instantpot.com Use code JP for extra savings

Journey Bar – plant-based food bars, www.journeybar.com (use coupon code johnpierre)

Now Foods – quality supplements, foods, essential oils, teas, and much more; many Now products are available at www.nowfoods.com

Numi Tea – organic high-quality tea varieties, www.numitea.com

NuTru – quality vegan supplements, available at www.nutru.com

Organic Food Bar – plant-based food bars, www.organicfoodbar.com

Power Systems – quality fitness products; available at www.johnpierre.com: click Shop, Power Systems

Plantiva – quality nutritional suppliments; available at plantiva.com

Pro-Tec Athletics – quality first aid support products and more; available at www.pro-tecathletics.com

Rebel Desk – quality stand-up desks and work treadmills available at www.rebeldesk.com

RevGear–quality martial arts and fitness gear; available at revgear.com

RumbleRoller – high quality foam rollers; available at www.rumbleroller.com

SoDelicious – vegan cultured coconut milk, nut milks, nut-based ice creams, and much more, sodeliciousdairyfree.com

Solute ions – electrolytes, trace mineral drops; available at www.johnpierre.com; click Shop, Solute ions

Sunwarrior – plant-based protein powders, www.sunwarrior.com

Thorlos – quality socks; available at www.thorlo.com

Tofurky– plant based foods and recipes, www.tofurky.com

Trainingmask.com–quality endurance products and more.

Tribest – quality food dehydrators, juicers, and personal blenders; available at www.johnpierre.com: click Shop, then choose Tribest Dehydrator, Juice Extractor, or Personal Blender

Ultraslide – quality slide boards and more, www.ultraslide.com

Vega – quality protein powders and nutritional support, myvega.com

22DaysNutrition.com –quality plant based food bars.

Magazines

American Vegan – americanvegan.org

NAVS: Vegetarian Voice – navs.org

Thrive Magazine – mythrivemag.com

Vegan Health and Fitness – veganhealthandfitnessmag.com

VegNews – vegnews.com

VegWorld Magazine –www.vegworldmag.com

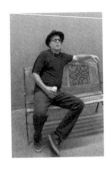 **Special thanks to JVonD, a great guy who played the "bad guy."**

JVonD Productions at JVonD.com

Photo credits: Alan Raz, John Pierre, Marina Alexander
So Delicious Dairy Free photos pages 119 and 121 used with permission.
Cover design: Victoria Hart
Back cover design: Victoria Hart
Cover photos: Alan Raz, John Pierre

Endnotes

Chapter 1: Programmed Violence

Glorified Violence on Display

1. Gardner, David. 12 Little-Known Ways that Television Stifles Spiritual Awakening. 9/8/2014 Waking Times. http://www.wakingtimes.com/2014/09/08/12-little-known-ways-television-stifles-spiritual-awakening/ (accessed September 10, 2014).

2. United States Department of Labor. Bureau of Labor Statistics. American Time Use Survey Summery. June 18, 2014. http://www.bls.gov/news.release/atus.nr0.htm (accessed September 10, 2014).

3. Andersen RE, Crespo CJ, Bartlett SJ, Cheskin LJ, Pratt M: Relationship of physical activity and television watching with body weight and level of fatness among children: results from the Third National Health and Nutrition Examination Survey. *JAMA* 279:938–942, 1998.

4. "Media Violence: Facts and Statistics." Media Education Foundation. http://www.jacksonkatz.com/PDF/ChildrenMedia.pdf (accessed March 20, 2014); "The Psychological Effects of Children's Movies." Association for Natural Psychology. http://www.winmentalhealth.com/childrens_movies_media_effects.php (accessed November 25, 2013). Andalo, Debbie."Child aggression linked to violent media." Society Guardian. http://www.guardian.co.uk/society/2005/feb/18/health.uknews (accessed October 19, 2012).

5. Clark, Laura. "Cartoon violence 'makes children more aggressive." http://www.dailymail.co.uk/news/article-1159766/Cartoon-violence-makes-children-aggressive.html (accessed September 19, 2013).

6. Cantor, Joanne. Ph.D. "The Psychological Effects of Media Violence on Children and Adolescents." http:// yourmindonmedia.com/wp-content/uploads/ media_violence_paper.pdf (accessed November 25, 2013).

7. Singer, M. I., Slovak, K., Frierson, T., & York, P. (1998). "Viewing preferences, symptoms of psychological trauma, and violent behaviors among children who watch television." *Journal of the American Academy of Child and Adolescent Psychiatry*, 37, 1041-1048.

8. Crane, Misti. "Kids' aggressive behavior tied to TV violence in studies." http://www.dispatch.com/content/stories/local/ 2013/02/18/kids-aggressive-behavior-tied-to-tv-violence-in-studies.html (accessed September 20, 2013)

9. Lemish, D. (1997). "The school as a wrestling arena: The modeling of a television series." Communication: European Journal of Communication Research, 22 (4), 395- 418.

10. Huesmann, L. Rowell. "Imitation and the Effects of Observing Media Violence on Behavior." February 11, 2003.http://www.rcgd.isr.umich.edu/aggr/articles Huesmann2005.Huesmann.Imitation&theeffectsofobservingmedi aviolonbehavr.Imitation,humandev&culture.pdf (accessed November 25, 2013).

11. Molitor, F., & Hirsch, K. W. (1994). "Children's toleration of real-life aggression after exposure to media violence: A replication of the Drabman and Thomas studies." *Child Study Journal*, 24, 191-207. http://mediaviolence.org/media-video-violence-addiction-research/research-archives/molitor-f-hirsch-k-w-1994-childrens-toleration-of-real-life-aggression-after-exposure-to-media-violence-a-replication-of-the-drabman-and-thomas-studies-child-study-journal-24-3-191 (accessed November 25, 2013).

12. Mullin, C.R., & Linz, D. (1995). "Desensitization and resensitization to violence against women: Effects of exposure to sexually violent films on judgments of domestic violence

victims." *Journal of Personality and Social Psychology*, 69, 449-459.

13. Key, Wilson Bryan. *Subliminal Seduction*. New Jersey: Prentice-Hall Inc. 1972

14. Key, Wilson Bryan. *The Age of Manipulation: The con in confidence, the sin in sincere.* New York, NY. Henry Holt and Co. 1989.

15. "The FCC's Investigation of 'Subliminal Techniques." From the Sublime to the Absurd. Press Statement September 19, 2000. http://transition.fcc.gov/Speeches/Furchtgott_Roth/2000/sphfr011.html (accessed November 26,2013) FCC Press Statement March 9, 2001. http://transition.fcc.gov/Speeches/Tristani/Statements/2001/stgt123.html (accessed November 26, 2013).

Recreation or "Wreck-Creation?"

1. Lemmens JS, Valkenburg PM, and Peter J. "The effects of pathological gaming on aggressive behavior." *Journal of Youth and Adolescence.* Jan;401 (1):38-47 http://www.ncbi.nlm.nih.gov/pubmed/20549320 (accessed November 26, 2013).

2. Anderson CA, et al. "Violent video game effects on aggression, empathy, and prosocial behavior in eastern and western countries: a meta-analytic review." *Psychological Bulletin.* March 2010; 136 (2): 151-173 http://www.ncbi.nlm.nih.gov/pubmed/20192553 (accessed November 26, 2013).

3. Frölich J, Lehmkuhl G, Döpfner M. "Computer games in childhood and adolescence: relations to addictive behavior, ADHD, and aggression." *Z Kinder Jugendpsychiatr Psychother.* 2009 Sep; 37(5):393-402; quiz 403-4. http://www.ncbi.nlm.nih.gov/pubmed/20549320 (accessed November 26, 2013).

4. Bagot, Martin. "GTA 5 torture row: Teachers slam scenes of extreme violence in most expensive game ever made." http://www.mirror.co.uk/lifestyle/staying-in/video-games/gta-5-torture-row-teachers-2278689 (accessed September 20, 2013)

5. Nayak, Malathi. "Take Two's Grand Theft Auto roars off starting line with US$800m debut." http://www.scmp.com/business/companies/article/1312919/take-twos-grand-theft-auto-roars-starting-line-us800m-debut (accessed September 20, 2013)

6. Bagot, Martin. "GTA 5 torture row: Teachers slam scenes of extreme violence in most expensive game ever made." http://www.mirror.co.uk/lifestyle/staying-in/video-games/gta-5-torture-row-teachers-2278689 (accessed September 20, 2013)

Inflammatory Lyrics

1-3. Key, Wilson Bryan. *Subliminal Seduction*. New Jersey: Prentice-Hall Inc. 1972

4. Polcari A, Rabi K, Bolger E, and Teicher MH. "Parental verbal affection and verbal aggression in childhood differently influence psychiatric symptoms and wellbeing in young adulthood." November 20, 2013. Published ahead of print. http://www.ncbi.nlm.nih.gov/pubmed/24268711 (accessed November 26, 2013).

5. Martin SC, et al. "Exposure to degrading versus non degrading music lyrics and sexual behavior among youth." *Pediatrics*. 2006 Aug; 118(2) http://www.ncbi.nlm.nih.gov/pubmed/16882784 (accessed November 26, 2013).

XXX Seeds of Destruction

1. Ybarra ML, et al. "X-rated material and perpetration of sexually aggressive behavior among children and adolescents: is there a link?" *Aggressive Behavior*. 2011 Jan-Feb; 37(1): 1-18 http://www.ncbi.nlm.nih.gov/pubmed/21046607 (accessed November 26, 2013).

2. Morgenstern, Madeleine. "Steubenville Rape Trial: High School Football Players Found Guilty of Raping Drunken 16-Year-Old Girl, Sentenced to At Least 1 Year in Juvenile Jail." http://www.theblaze.com/stories/2013/03/17/steubenville-rape-trial-high-school-football-players-found-guilty-of-raping-drunken-16-year-old-girl/ (accessed November 30, 2013).

3. "Teenager 'who killed herself after pictures of her sexual assault went online' marched in Obama's 2008 inaugural parade." http://www.dailymail.co.uk/news/article-2309162/Audrie-Pott-case-Teenage-girl-killed-sexually-assaulted-boys-marched-Obamas-2008-inaugural-parade.html (accessed November 30, 2013)

4. Bridges AJ, at al. "Aggression and sexual behavior in best-selling pornography videos: a content analysis update." *Violence Against Women.* 2010 Oct; 16 (10): 1065-85 http://www.ncbi.nlm.nih.gov/pubmed/20980228 (accessed November 26, 2013).

5. Wright PJ. "U.S. males and pornography, 1973-2010: consumption, predictors, correlates." *Journal of Sex Research.* 2013; 50 (1) 60-71 http://www.ncbi.nlm.nih.gov/pubmed/22126160 (accessed November 26, 2013).

Lost Brain Function

1. Schauss, at al. "A Critical Analysis of the Diets of Chronic Juvenile Offenders: Part 2." *Orthomolecular Psychiatry*, Volume 8, No. 4, 1979, Pp. 222-226. http://orthomolecular.org/library/jom/1979/pdf/1979-v08n04-p222.pdf

2. Sutliff, Usha. "Nutrition Key to Aggressive Behavior." USC News.http://www.usc.edu/uscnews/stories/10773.html (accessed November 26, 2013).

3. Werbach, Melvyn R. "Nutritional Influences on Aggressive Behavior." *Journal of Orthomolecular Medicine* Vol.7, No.1, 1995. http://orthomolecular.org/library/articles/webach.shtml (accessed November 26, 2013).

4. Kitahara M. "Dietary trypotophan ratio and homicide in Western and Southern Europe." *Journal of Orthomolecular Medicine* 1(1):13-6, 1986.

Chapter 2: Identifying Malicious Intent

Predator Tools that Smother Intuition

1. McAllister, Sue. "Jury Convicts Twin Brothers in Date Rape Drugging Case." http://articles.latimes.com/1998/jun/18/local/me-61130 (accessed September 19, 2013) (accessed September 19,2013); Ritz, Erica. "Horrifying: Australian Woman Gang Raped in Dubai–Then Jailed 8 months for Sex Outside Marriage." http://www.theblaze.com/stories/2013/05/13/horrifying-australian-woman-gang-raped-in-dubai-then-jailed-for-8-months-for-sex-outside-marriage/# (acessed September 17, 2013)

2. Friedman, Ann. "When Rape Goes Viral." Newsweek. July 7, 2013. http://mag.newsweek.com/2013/07/24/when-rape-goes-viral.html (accessed March 24, 2014).

Retaining Unearned Trust

1. Ellis, Ralph. "San Antonio officer charged in patrol car sex assault." CNN Justice. November 25, 2013.http://www.cnn.com/2013/11/25/justice/san-antonio-officer-sex-assault/index.html?hpt=hp_t2 (accessed November 25, 2013).

2. Sattiewhite, Travis. "California officer accused of sexually assaulting 6 women." CNN Justice. February 26, 2013.http://www.cnn.com/2013/02/26/justice/california-officer-rape/index.html (accessed November 25, 2013).

Online Romeo's

1. Walberg, Matthew. "Man who used online dating site convicted of assault." Chicago Tribune. November 9, 2010.

http://articles.chicagotribune.com/2010-11-09/news/ct-met-match-com-rape-20101109_1_sexual-assault-judge-acquits-match-com (accessed March 24, 2014); Muir, David. "2009: Jeffrey Marsalis Speaks Publicly for First Time." ABC News. July 15, 2009. http://abcnews.go.com/Primetime/match-serial-rapist-jeffrey-marsalis-speaks-publicly/story?id=8069223 (accessed March 24, 2014).

Creepy Stalkers

1. Victim Survival Stalking Handbook. "Stalking and Criminal Threats." http://www.stalkingalert.com/VictimSurvivalHandbook.pdf (accessed March 20, 2014).

Chapter 4: Protecting Our Children

Family Escape Drills

1. U. S. Department of Justice Office of Justice Programs, Bureau of Justice Statistics. Victimization During Household Burglary, September 2010. http://www.bjs.gov/content/pub/ascii/vdhb.txt (accessed May 2, 2014).

Chapter 5: Back-Stabbing Industries

Tricked into Guzzling Misery

1. Adams, Carol. "Dairy is a Feminist Issue." September 21, 2012. http://caroljadams.blogspot.com/2012/09/dairy-is-feminist-issue.html (accessed March 20, 2014).

2. "How to Artificially Inseminate Cows and Heifers." http://m.wikihow.com/Artificially-Inseminate-Cows-and-Heifers (accessed March 20, 2014).

3. McDougall, John."Diet-Induced Precocious Puberty." The McDougall Newsletter (December 1997). http://

drmcdougall.com/newsletter/nov_dec97.html (accessed March 24, 2014).

4. Chen J.-C., Shao Z.-M., Sheikh M. S., Hussain A., Leroith D., Roberts C. T. and Fontana J. A. (1994), "Insulin-like growth factor-binding protein enhancement of insulin-like growth factor-i (IGF-I)- mediated DNA synthesis and IGF-I binding in a human breast carcinoma cell line," *Journal of Cell Physiology*, 158: 69–78. doi: 10. 1002/jcp. 1041580100; Li, Xiao-Su, Chen, Jian-Chyi, Sheikh, M. Saeed, Shao, Zhi-Ming, Fontana, Joseph A., "Ritinoic Acid Inhibition of Insulin-like Growth Factor I Stimulation of c-fosmRNA Levels in a Breast Carcinoma Cell Line," *Experimental Cell Research*, March 1994, 211(1). Duggan C, Wang CY, Neuhouser ML, Xiao L, Smith AW, Reding KW, Baumgartner RN, Baumgartner KB, Bernstein L, Ballard-Barbash R, McTiernan A, "Associations of insulin-like growth factor and insulin-like growth factor binding protein-3 with mortality in women with breast cancer," *International Journal of Cancer*, 2012, National Center for Biotechnology Information. http://www.ncbi.nlm.nih.gov/pubmed/22847383 (accessed March 24, 2014); Gallagher, Emily and LeRoith, Derek, "The Proliferating Role of Insulin and Insulin-Like Growth Factors in Cancer," *Trends in Endocrinology Metabolism*, National Center for Biotechnology Information, http://www.ncbi.nlm.nih.gov/pmc/articles/PMC2949481/?tool=pmcentrez (accessed March 24, 2014).

5. Campbell, T. Colin, and Campbell, Thomas M. The China Study: The Most Comprehensive Study of Nutrition Ever Conducted and the Startling Implications for Diet, Weight Loss and Long-Term Health. Dallas, TX: BenBella Books, 2005.

Chapter 6: Are You Fueling Yourself or Fooling Yourself?

Reclaiming Our Taste-buds and Brain Chemistry

1. Lisle, Douglas J. and Goldhamer, Alan, *The Pleasure Trap*, Summertown, TN: Healthy Living Publications, 2003;

Chapter 8: Prepared Resistance

1. "911 Dispatcher Tells Woman About To Be Sexually Assaulted There Are No Cops To Help Her Due To Budget Cuts." CBS Seattle, May 23, 2013: http://seattle.cbslocal.com/2013/05/23/911-dispatcher-tells-woman-about-to-be-sexually-assaulted-there-are-no-cops-to-help-her-due-to-budget-cuts/ (accessed November 26, 2013)

Understanding "Crime Scene Number 2"

1. Strong, Sanford. *Strong On Defense: Survival rules to protect you and your family from crime.* New York: Simon and Schuster, 1996.

2. Barr, Meghan and Sheeran, Thomas J. "Women held Captive in Ohio endured lonely, dark lives: kidnap suspect due in court Thursday." StarTribune May 9, 2013.http://www.startribune.com/206564831.html (accessed September 26, 2013)

Never Give Up

1. Prather, Shannon. "Anoka woman who fought back during knife attack tells others to "Fight Like a Girl." http://www.startribune.com/local/north/211075781.html (acessed September 25, 2013).

About the Authors

John Pierre is a nutrition and fitness consultant who has devoted more than 25 years to improving the lives of others through his expertise in the areas of nutrition, fitness, women's empowerment, green living, and cognitive enhancement. A dedicated activist, John works with people of all ages promoting the benefits of a plant-based diet, stress reduction, and physical fitness, and the importance of compassion in life. He is widely recognized in the area of geriatrics for enhancing cognitive function in our senior population. John has been lecturing for more than 20 years at various venues that reach thousands of people. His website, www.johnpierre.com, has served as a vital resource in helping people become active in their communities by taking just five minutes to voice their thoughts on important environmental, humanitarian, and animal rights issues.

Marina Alexander is a freelance writer and researcher with a passion for fitness, nutrition, health, and women's empowerment. This is her second writing contribution.